W9-BFF-173

Also by **MARK S. GOLD,** M.D.

The Good News About Panic, Anxiety and Phobias
The 800-COCAINE Book
The Good News About Depression
The Facts About Drugs and Alcohol
Wonder Drugs

THE GOOD NEWS ABOUT DRUGS AND ALCOHOL

THE GOOD NEWS ABOUT DRUGS AND ALCOHOL

Curing, Treating and Preventing Substance Abuse in the New Age of Biopsychiatry

MARK S. GOLD, M.D.

Villard Books New York 1991

 Published in the United States by Villard Books, a division of Random House, Inc., New York, and simultaneously in Canada by Random House of Canada Limited, Toronto.

Although the case histories in this book are accurate, the names and identifying characteristics of the persons described have been changed to protect their privacy.

Library of Congress Cataloging-in-Publication Data
Gold, Mark S.
The good news about drugs and alcohol: curing, treating and preventing substance abuse in the new age of biopsychiatry/by Mark S. Gold, M.D.
p. cm.
Includes bibliographical references and index.
ISBN 0-394-58949-1
1. Drug abuse—Treatment. 2. Alcoholism—Treatment.
3. Biological psychiatry. I. Title.
RC564.G65 1991 616.86—dc20 90-50661

BOOK DESIGN BY CATHRYN S. AISON

Manufactured in the United States of America
9 8 7 6 5 4 3 2

FIRST EDITION

To my mentors:
George Aghajanian, M.D., Robert Byck, M.D.,
Herbert Kleber, M.D., D. Eugene Redmond, M.D.,
and Steven Zornetzer, Ph.D.

ACKNOWLEDGMENTS

I am especially grateful to my collaborators, colleagues, and patients at Fair Oaks Hospital and Yale University.

For their contributions to this book, my sincerest thanks go to A. Carter Pottash, M.D., Dan Montopoli, Janice Finn Gold, M.Ed., M.P.H., Ron Schaumburg, Willie Hayden, Larry Chilnick, Barbara Capone, and Mary Hallock.

CONTENTS

INTRODUCTION

As a father, I want my children to grow up happy and healthy, to reach the fullest flowering of their potential. As an American, I want my country to thrive. As a human being, I want to see an end to suffering wherever it is found. And as a physician—a psychiatrist specializing in treating substance abuse—I want to treat people with education before they are addicted. For our patients, I want them to be free of their dependencies, whatever form that dependency takes.

If I were to wake up tomorrow and find that all drugs had been eliminated, that all current addicts had been cured and all future addictions thwarted, I would be the happiest man in the world, and I would gladly find something else to do! That's not likely to happen, though. My job is, unfortunately, very secure. That's why I devote as much energy as I can to spreading the word about drugs. We all know the bad news about drugs—this book represents the good news.

This book also represents a tribute to the countless number of individuals who fought the battles against drugs in their lives, in their families, in their schools, and in their communities. While their victories have been impressive, much work remains

—especially in our cities, where drug use continues to be a major problem.

We need a new drug war specifically tailored to overcoming drugs in areas that have largely resisted our best efforts. I want this book to serve as a guide both to continue our successful efforts and to help evolve new strategies in the years ahead. Drug abuse is a problem that we can never ignore.

Throughout my entire professional life I've focused on the problem of drug use in one form or another. At medical school I noticed that students used amphetamines—"speed"—to help them stay awake while cramming for exams. Curious about the effects of these drugs on memory, I conducted a study and found that, if Joe Medschool crams while in a drugged state, he will also have to use speed—and in the same dose—during the test as well, or he won't be able to come up with the answers. This phenomenon is called the "state dependency of memory."

Later, during residency training at Yale, I studied the new and revolutionary science of neurobiology, which explores the connections between biology and psychiatry. At one point I observed that monkeys suffering from a chemically or electrically induced "anxiety" state acted just like human beings in the throes of heroin withdrawal. That insight led me to explore the use of a drug called clonidine as a way to block the symptoms of withdrawal from opiates. Now clonidine is used as a routine part of successful detoxification treatment of opiate addicts and even children of addicts. I'll have more to say about clonidine and other new treatments in Chapter Thirteen.

In 1978, I moved to Fair Oaks Hospital in Summit, New Jersey. There, along with some of my talented colleagues from Yale and other schools, we applied the lessons we had learned about the biological aspects of psychiatry, or biopsychiatry as it came to be known. We focused on the physical causes of such illnesses as depression, eating disorders, and addiction. Our goal was, and still is, to return psychiatry to its origin as a medical discipline, and to use the tools of medicine—physical examination, diagnostic techniques, pharmaceutical therapies —in the most effective ways to help our patients get better. In

Chapter Three I'll explain how biopsychiatry has revolutionized the treatment of substance abuse disorders.

During the last decade, the research we've done at Fair Oaks in New Jersey and in Florida has contributed vastly to our understanding of the nature and treatment of addictions. In 1983, Fair Oaks launched the 800-COCAINE Helpline, now a 24-hour-a-day telephone service. We gave callers accurate information about a "new" drug, cocaine, sent them information pamphlets and books about substance abuse, and suggested referrals for treatment; in turn, they helped us by answering questions that allowed us to track national trends in substance abuse. Some of the information in this book is based on several of 800-COCAINE's surveys.

Another avenue of biopsychiatric research led to the discovery that cocaine depletes the brain's supply of the neurotransmitter dopamine, needed to carry important signals from one cell to another. While this research was exciting in its own right, we took it a step further and developed a medical treatment for cocaine addicts. We found that a medication called bromocriptine helps replace those neurotransmitters and thus blocks the symptoms of cocaine withdrawal. Use of bromocriptine can be a vital step in ridding cocaine users of their addiction.

In addition to my work with patients and in the lab, I have used whatever free time I could find during the last 15 years to speak to my fellow physicians and to the public about the drug problem. In recent years I have been privileged to serve as an adviser, first to Ronald Reagan's White House office of drug policy and then to President Bush's former "drug czar," William Bennett. And I look forward to helping the new "drug czar," Bob Martinez, in any way I can. I publish articles in medical journals and the lay press, write books, and serve as a board member of national prevention organizations (Parent's Resource Institute for Drug Education (PRIDE) and the American Council for Drug Education)—anything I can to hammer the point home, including helping the Partnership for a Drug Free America in its educational efforts.

I can say with certainty—and with a forgivable degree of pride—that the nation is making tremendous progress in its fight against drugs. One goal of this book is to highlight examples of success and to describe ways of building on those triumphs in the home, school, and community so we can keep the momentum going.

THE GOOD NEWS ABOUT DRUGS AND ALCOHOL

CHAPTER ONE

Today's War Against Drugs

"I was supposed to go to a movie with a guy. But before we got there he wanted us to smoke dope. 'Why?' I said. 'Because it'll make the movie more fun.' I said, 'That's just fake fun. If going to the movies with me isn't enough fun for you, then I don't want to go.' "

"What happened?" I asked.

"I dumped him," she said.

Another girl spoke up, "I don't use drugs because I saw what they did to my brother. He used to be okay—you know, the typical pain-in-the-neck older brother, but mostly he was okay. Then he changed. He'd fight all the time, with me, with my parents. He'd stay in his room and never come down for dinner. My parents didn't know what to do. They never even liked to talk about him. They kept making excuses. They didn't know what was going on. But I knew. He didn't try to hide it from me. He just scared me, told me to keep quiet or else. Then one day he didn't come home. No phone call, no message, he just disappeared. I haven't seen him since. I'm not letting that happen to me. I'm gonna be a lawyer and make a million dollars a year. I can't afford to blow my brains out on crack."

"I'm worried for the little kids," said one 11-year-old boy. "My nephew—he's only seven—he said he was playing at the playground and some guy came up and pulled a bag of white stuff out of the garbage can. Man, if I catch anyone trying to mess up my nephew, I'm gonna mess *them* up." His classmates cheered.

As I stood there in front of his middle-school assembly, I couldn't help thinking back to the early 1980s. When I spoke to students then, their attitude was skeptical and full of scorn. I remember one girl challenged me by saying, "Marijuana can't be all that bad. My mom and dad said they smoked a lot, and they turned out okay. So will I." Another student remarked, "My dad drinks scotch every night and my mom smokes a pack of cigarettes a day. Who are they to tell me doing drugs is wrong?"

Today, though, at the end of my talk the kids cheer. They aren't cheering for me, though, they're cheering for themselves. And they're cheering for my message.

After decades of looking the other way, after years of disastrous efforts at decriminalization and legalization, after being told to "drop out and tune in," after our medical experts falsely compared cocaine to chocolate, after millions of lives have been ruined—America has finally recognized its most formidable enemy: drugs. To protect its people and its families, we've declared war—and the good news is, we're winning.

Consider:

- The number of current drug users *fell* from 23 million to 12.9 million—a drop of 44 percent—between 1985 and 1990.
- In 1988, the number of people who had used drugs within the previous 12 months also steadily declined from 37 million to 28 million. In 1990 this figure dropped to 27 million.
- In 1985 there were 5.8 million current users of cocaine; five years later, that number was cut—to 1.6 million.
- From 1988 to 1990 there was a 26 percent decrease in the number of cocaine-related emergency room visits.
- Marijuana use is at its lowest point since 1972.

- In 1985, 18 million claimed to have smoked pot within the previous month; in 1988, only 12 million made such a claim.
- America's consumption of liquor is at its lowest point in 30 years.
- Drug rehabilitation centers are half-full and many are closing.
- Drug use is no longer considered "normal."

Surprised? I'm not. Twelve years ago Dr. Herbert Kleber, my mentor at Yale University, and I predicted that if this country could harness its medical knowledge, its public relations skills, its mass media talents, and its educational drive, we could win the war on drugs. Our predictions are coming true.

There is of course a great deal more to learn and do, but we do know one critical fact: *antidrug strategies work.* Education can be as powerful as any treatment! We know what message we should communicate and how to communicate it. We can spot the people on the brink of disaster, throw them a lifeline, and return them to a healthy and happy life. We can identify people in need, intervene, and treat them in their community without losing jobs or homes. We have strategies that can work against drug abuse in the office, at school, at home, and even in our streets. These strategies are, in a nutshell, *The Good News About Drugs and Alcohol.*

Here are a few more examples of America's new resolve:

- Realizing that the police alone couldn't stop the drugs in their neighborhood, Jean Veldwyk and Norm Chamberlain created the South Seattle Crime Prevention Council (SSCPC). They set up a hotline to deal with such problems as drug dealing and gang activity. Within 18 months police closed down approximately 1,000 crack houses—400 of which had been reported on the SSCPC hotline. As Ms. Veldwyk put it, neighborhood residents have become the "eyes and ears of the community."
- The Fairlawn Coalition in Washington, D.C., is a group formed by citizens who got tired of the traffic jams caused by drug buyers cruising their neighborhood. Volunteers wearing bright orange baseball caps are equipped with radios, video

cameras, and binoculars to spot, report, and record drug activity. Their strategy has worked; the dealers disappeared, and so have their customers.

- Concerned about their native city, two lifelong residents of Portland, Oregon, founded a program they call Self-Enhancement, Inc. SEI identifies kids who are at risk of getting into trouble with drugs and provides alternatives to involvement in gangs or drugs. Since the program began, some 700 youngsters have learned to improve their academic and communication skills—as well as their self-respect.

People have gotten the message: Get involved and don't wait for someone else to take the initiative. Properly armed with facts, people have made the difference.

Still, much work remains. Drug dealing continues to be a huge and powerful multinational operation. The Drug Enforcement Agency (DEA) estimates that a hundred billion dollars' worth of illicit drugs are sold every year in this country alone—twice what we spend on oil. A legitimate corporation doing that much business would place high in the Top Ten of the Fortune 500 companies. Worldwide, the total is probably close to $500 billion.

Further, one out of 12 Americans—21 million people—say they smoke marijuana on occasion. In 1990, there were an estimated 15 to 18 million people classified as alcohol-dependent. Another 3 million use cocaine—with some estimates labelling 1.7 million users as "hard-core." While casual drug use has decreased, deaths from cocaine and heroine have increased by 10.7 and 5.8 percent respectively between 1988 and 1989. There are perhaps half a million heroin addicts. As one Treasury Department official observed, "Any industry with 25 million American consumers can support an enormous empire."

But the number of users isn't the only problem. The users are getting younger. Responding to a *Weekly Reader* survey, kids in the sixth grade reported feeling pressure to try drugs—pressure not from some stranger lurking in the school yard, but from their own classmates. Roughly 60 percent of marijuana users now report that their first experience with drugs came between the sixth and ninth grades. In fact, a Detroit Little League team had to disband because the players were more interested in smoking crack than playing ball.

No one is immune. Drug abusers can be found among the ranks of corporate executives, lawyers, even doctors and nurses. A police chief in Massachusetts—a noted antidrug activist—was accused of stealing cocaine from the police evidence room. He later admitted he had used cocaine every day for five years. Seventy percent of all drug users are employed! Drugs are clearly an "equal opportunity destroyer."

Drug use doesn't just affect those who inhale the smoke or stick a needle in their arm. It affects parents, spouses, children, relatives, employers, friends. A nationwide *Wall Street Journal*/NBC News poll in 1989 found that the lives of three out of four Americans had been touched by drugs. When the Reverend George Clements in Chicago asked those in his congregation who had a drug-addicted relative to stand, all 800 members rose.

Also in 1989, in a poll conducted annually by *The New York Times*/CBS News, 64 percent of those interviewed identified drugs as the nation's leading problem—ahead of nuclear war, pollution, or crime. That figure represented a huge jump from the previous year, when only 20 percent considered drugs our biggest headache. In a survey of teenagers by the Gallup organization, 54 percent named drug abuse as the biggest problem facing their generation—double the number who felt that way ten years before. And a *USA Today* survey in October 1989 found that 88 percent of Americans now believe the drug crisis is worse than most people realize, and that it is *not* the product of media hype. In March 1991, pollster Robert Teeter cited a study in which, by a ratio of four to one, the American people thought the drug problem was getting worse.

In some respects, these numbers are horrifying. They reveal a pattern of widespread drug use, addiction suffering, and fear. But I look at those numbers and see *good* news. For one thing, they mean the antidrug message is getting through and that

American attitudes are changing. For another, now that we've admitted there's a problem, we can get on with the task of correcting it.

Good news turned up in the 1990 National Institute of Drug Abuse (NIDA) survey of high school seniors. The survey found that:

- Drug use among seniors is at its lowest level since 1975.
- In 1985 nearly 30 percent admitted to using at least one illegal drug within the past month, while in 1990 this number dropped to slightly over 17 percent.
- From 1985 to 1990, the proportion of seniors who have used cocaine at least once in their lifetimes dropped from 17.3 percent to 9.4 percent.
- The percentage of seniors who believed that smoking marijuana posed a great risk has risen from 35 percent in 1978 to over 77 percent in 1990.
- Between 1981 and 1990, the percentage of seniors who disapproved of adults using cocaine even once or twice increased from 74 percent to 91.5 percent.

In September 1990, The Partnership for a Drug-Free America released data from the largest attitudinal survey on illegal drugs that found teenage use of marijuana declined 27 percent and teenage use of cocaine dropped 44 percent from 1989 to 1990.

Clearly our high school students are getting the message.

Writing in the *New England Journal of Medicine,* drug experts Drs. Frank H. Gawin and E. H. Ellinwood, Jr., observed that "There have been unprecedented public representations of cocaine's dangers. Perhaps because of this new awareness, the incidence of first-time cocaine use has just begun to decline." Education can be a potent preventative treatment.

Let's look at that trend in graphic form.

The Graph on page 9 illustrates tens of thousands of student responses to three questions posed each year between 1975 and 1990, concerning:

1. **Availability:** the percentage of students responding that cocaine is "fairly easy" or "very easy" to get;

2. **Perceived Risk:** the percentage of students saying that

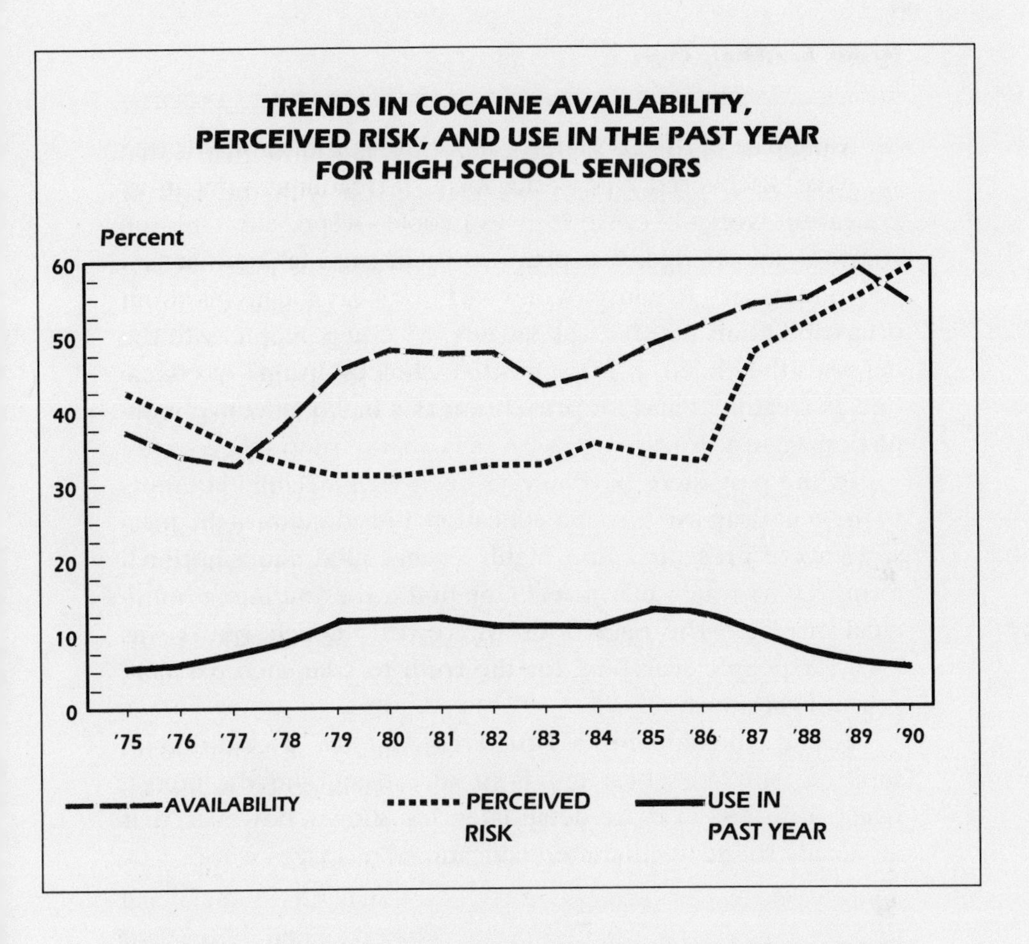

there is a "great risk" of harm if people take cocaine once or twice; and

3. Use in the Past Year: the percentage of students who have used cocaine within the last year.

The curves of these three lines outline an exciting piece of good news. When students are unaware of the risks of cocaine, use of the drug soars; but when they understand the dangers, use plummets—*even though the drug is easy to get.*

Now that most people see drugs as a tremendous threat, they are demanding that things change. With the strength of their numbers, they are pressuring federal and local governments to take action. They are drawing on the resources of their schools and communities to spread the message. In fact, when asked if they would be willing to bear some kind of tax increase to finance the fight against drugs, 63 percent of those surveyed in *The Wall Street Journal* poll said yes.

A big part of the good news about drugs and alcohol is that we have discovered a powerful form of treatment: education. Education works because it gives people—especially children—a tool, knowledge, that prevents them from taking that first step on the road to abuse. When we blow away the myths about drugs and point out the real dangers, we equip people with the defenses they need to make positive choices. I think of education as treatment and for prevention as a highly effective inoculation against drugs.

In the past there have always been well-meaning attempts to prevent drug use through education. But sometimes the messages were presented in a highly exaggerated and emotional form: "Don't touch marijuana! One puff turns you into a homicidal maniac!" The risks of drugs are real enough, but it was hard for people searching for the truth to take such extreme warnings seriously.

The Partnership for a Drug-Free America, a coalition of some of America's best minds in advertising and the media, which I discuss in more detail later, has shown, however, that medically sound, well-crafted educational messages work.

The Tools in the Fight Against Drugs

There are three elements that have contributed to our success over drugs thus far: people, information, and attitudes.

People During World War II, the population pulled together to support the war effort. Today the enemy is alcohol, not the Axis; narcotics, not Nazis. But when people focus their energies in a collective effort, the result will be the same: victory on all fronts. At every level of society, people are becoming involved with the movement away from drugs. As you can tell from the examples I've already cited, indifference and denial have given way to concern and commitment.

Parents are waking up to the fact that their children are in danger, and are taking steps to protect them. Schoolteachers and administrators realize the critical role they play in preventing drug use and are building an antidrug message into the curriculum at the earliest grade levels. Community leaders donate their services, expertise, and facilities in support of antidrug efforts.

Corporate executives and industry leaders know that sponsoring employee-assistance programs and antidrug campaigns helps not just their workers but their bottom lines as well. Sensing the social trend away from drinking, hotel owners have begun to take out their liquor bars and replace them with food-service areas. Advertisers and media owners disperse free antidrug messages through television, radio, and print. Government officials and civil servants, from presidents to police officers, attempt to devise and enforce laws to control the supply of drugs and punish those who distribute or use them.

Information Another weapon is information. Those who fight the drug scourge rely on facts—hard, accurate facts—to wage their campaign.

Years ago I conducted studies that proved the addictive power of cocaine, that deepened our understanding of the ways chemicals affect bodies, personalities, and perceptions, and that showed how drugs could ruin people's lives. In the early 1980s, I spoke at schools, churches, and professional meetings, sometimes bringing along a recovering celebrity or athlete. For a while I felt as if I was one of a small group speaking out. Now, with scientific data to go along with the horror stories of ex-addicts, it is impossible to question the effects of cocaine. Countless others have reinforced and expanded upon my findings. Amazing new imaging devices allow us to watch the human brain in action—live and in color—as drugs take over. As this and other information is distributed around the world with extraordinary swiftness, the myths of the past are exposed and replaced with the realities of today. *We have learned more about the biology of addiction in the last ten years than in all the previous centuries combined.*

Of even greater significance, these facts have led to new treatments that allow even long-term addicts to kick their habits and remain drug-free for the rest of their lives. I get calls and cards from people I have treated who have been drug-free for ten years or more and from others who have been able to stop their drug use before professional treatment was necessary.

I believe that the solid information derived from my research and the research of others has played an important role in the current slowing of cocaine use. I also feel that access to the facts has made people aware of the dangers of all drugs. People now realize that the same "experts" who a few years ago declared cocaine to be safe or not yet proven dangerous were wrong—dead wrong. All drugs should be considered unsafe, or even deadly, until *proven* otherwise—not vice versa.

I have written this book as another weapon in the battle of information versus drugs. It contains as many hard facts as I could cram into it, facts I hope will prove useful to everyone.

Attitudes Here's another, and very critical, part of the good news about drugs and alcohol: Society's attitudes are undergoing a complete upheaval.

A quarter century ago, drug use emerged from the underground and became a part of mainstream culture. Users thought themselves "hip" or "cool." Movies, TV shows, books, and magazines depicted drugs as offering everything from a rip-roaring good time to profound insight into the universe. During the late 1970s cocaine was the big "in joke" on TV's *Saturday Night Live.* In a word, we used drugs, found them funny, and tolerated drug use.

Today, nobody's laughing anymore. People are fed up with death and destruction. They no longer stand idly by and watch as their neighborhoods, their families, and their dreams go up in smoke. They hate what is happening to the country, and they have begun to turn that hatred into a positive force against drugs.

In 1977, *Newsweek* observed that cocaine was being given out at fashionable cocktail parties along with the canapés and caviar. But in a dramatic reversal, the same magazine in 1986 compared the scourge of drugs to the Black Death. Even the editors of *Playboy* observed recently that the odds against surviving drug use were "much greater than we, or anyone else, would have believed" in the 1970s. The best message, the *Playboy* editors agreed, is still "Don't take drugs."

As Dr. Louis Sullivan, the Secretary of Health and Human Services, observed: "Attitudes *are* changing. And this is testimony to years of hard work by parents, educators, health care providers, employers, and religious leaders, as well as government efforts, to create a general social attitude that drug use is wrong and intolerable."

One reason for the change in society's attitude about cocaine is the speed with which its destructive effects become evident. While it might take years for alcohol to rot an alcoholic's liver, the destructive power of cocaine shows up much more quickly. A schoolteacher who starts using coke at the start of the semester may be gone by midterm. A football player on coke might go from being a star receiver at the start of the season to a fumbling, accident-prone embarrassment before the play-offs. Cocaine, with all the power and speed of time-lapse photography, has taught everyone about addictive illness.

Another helpful change of attitude emerged a couple of decades ago when we began to classify alcoholism and drug addiction as biological illnesses and not the result of some failure of morality or willpower. By shifting our perspective, and by recognizing that addiction has a biological basis, we have opened the door to new research and treatment possibilities. I'll focus more on that important subject in Chapter Four.

A landmark in the fight against substance abuse in general, and alcohol abuse in particular, occurred in 1990 when warning labels began to appear on every alcoholic beverage container. These labels state that drinking increases the risk of birth defects and health problems and that it impairs the ability to drive.

Even before the advent of the labels, we had evidence that the per capita consumption of alcohol is dropping. So is the rate of mortality due to cirrhosis of the liver and the incidence of alcohol-related traffic deaths. If the success of this educational effort comes anywhere close to the impact that the warnings on cigarette packages have had, I predict a big decline in the incidence of alcohol-related problems in this country. And that is *very* good news.

The Battlegrounds

Families Drug abuse is a family problem—a fact that the two national groups that I have worked closely with for almost a decade, The National Federation of Parents for a Drug-Free Youth (NFP) and the Parent's Resource Institute for Drug Education (PRIDE), realized from the beginning. As we'll see in the section on treatment, any substance abuse program that doesn't address family issues is doomed to fail. Fortunately, awareness of this fact has led to the creation of many effective family treatment programs and support groups. But whether out of love, lack of awareness, or willful blindness, many parents ignore signs of drug use among their children or other family members. Drugs are something the "other" kids do.

I believe the parental tendency toward self-delusion is changing. But we need to work harder to convince parents that no one is immune from drug abuse. We have the data to show parents that they have no reason to believe alcohol and drug abuse are "someone else's problem." Each day, we are learning more about specific risk factors, such as children who drop out of school, children of alcoholics, and children of drug users, that may make a child more vulnerable to drugs. The risk may even be higher if there is a sibling who uses drugs. If we can get the message across that sixth graders—kids just 11 or 12 years old—are being pressured to try drugs, parents will be more willing to launch the antidrug campaign at home. In Chapter Nine I'll offer some suggestions on how parents can help their children develop the right attitudes from the start.

Schools To me, the thought that a child can sit at her desk, look out the window, and witness a drug deal being consummated on the playground is shocking—and inexcusable.

I know I'm not alone in feeling this. Fortunately, many

school districts realize that teaching drug awareness is part of their responsibility. Innovative and aggressive drug programs have been woven into educational curricula from Washington State to Washington D.C. From kindergarten on, students are getting the message they desperately need to hear. What's more, schools are finding ways to provide drug-free after-school activities, including parties and athletics. To reinforce the message, they are developing—and enforcing—strict antidrug policies on campus.

Within the past few years, following the example set by New Jersey, a number of states have established drug-free school zones. These zones give notice that any drug use or sales occurring near schools will be punished much more severely than elsewhere in the community. Does it work? You better believe it. According to the director of security for the Newark, New Jersey, Board of Education, the zones resulted in a *50 percent decrease* in drug use in the schools within the first year.

In Chapter Ten we'll take a closer look at some of the model school drug programs around the country and describe the skills students learn for resisting drug pressure.

Workplaces A 1989 survey revealed that 64 percent of management executives now believe that substance abuse is the nation's most critical labor and employment problem. Drug use in the workplace exacts a terrible toll in low productivity, accidents, and poor product quality.

The chairman of General Motors once estimated that substance abuse costs the company over *one billion dollars a year* in treatment and worker absenteeism. One crack addict working for the auto maker told a reporter for *The New York Times:* "There's a madness out there. There are crack smokers sitting in offices making decisions and guys working on the line and running machines. And they don't believe they have a problem. It takes so long to learn. It's like blind men trying to lead blind men. They can't. So if you're blind, you better get yourself a dog."

Fortunately, business and industry are getting that "dog"—they know it's better to help employees conquer substance abuse and return to the job than to fire them and retrain new workers. Although the recession of 1991 has forced some companies to curtail health-care benefits, a substantial number of companies have added education, prevention, and treatment programs. The results, as we'll see in Chapter Eleven, are higher staff morale, better productivity—and a stronger bottom line.

One way to reduce drug use in the workplace is through testing. Already, more than half of the Fortune 500 companies have some form of drug-testing program. Some require all applicants to submit to urine tests before they will be considered for a position. Others periodically test people who work in certain areas, such as security, or whose job performance affects their safety and the safety of others. One company, SmithKline Beecham Clinical Laboratories, reported that 13 percent of their 1 million workers and job applicants tested positive for drug use during the first six months of 1990. While this figure remains unacceptably high, it is a significant improvement over 1987, when 18 percent tested positive. Harry Groome, the president of the company, attributed this decline to increased attention to drug use in the workplace. In Chapter Eleven I'll outline some of the techniques—and the controversies—of drug testing.

How Our Society Is Fighting Back

Grass-Roots Resistance Community groups, churches, and private citizens are striking back at drug dealers to reclaim their neighborhoods. Some people march against crack houses, barring would-be customers from getting to the door. Others open their homes to groups of young people, offering them drug-free activities and a place to socialize. In Dallas, Dorothy Davis, horrified by the drug-related death of a 12-year-old girl, organized her neighbors to form STOP Crime Watch. Similarly, Ruth Varnado and Queen Hyler of Milwaukee organized that city's Stop the Violence Movement. Such grass-roots resistance is extremely heartening and successful. (See Box on page 17.)

One Girl's Fight Against Drugs

"We're gonna move on you! You're gonna get violated!"

For a long time, Lacrista, 18 years old, endured such taunts and threats. The threats came from the girls who belonged to one of the many street gangs haunting the alleyways near her school on Chicago's South Side.

What had Lacrista done that so offended the gang? Had she tried to muscle in on their lucrative trade in illegal drugs? Had she violated one of the gang's many rules—tying her shoelaces the wrong way or wearing a jacket of the wrong color?

No. Lacrista had angered the gang because she refused to join them in selling drugs to her classmates. She was straight—and she wanted to stay that way.

In the eyes of the gang, Lacrista did everything wrong. She was a good student, active on the school's volleyball team and in after-school clubs. She had her eyes on the future and was looking forward to going to college so that she could become a teacher.

And she was smart. She knew drugs were nothing but trouble. She had seen firsthand the damage drugs can do. One of her brothers was in jail; another had been murdered three years earlier in a gang fight involving drugs. Many of her schoolmates were lost in a drug-induced fog.

One day as she left school she heard someone call out to her. She turned and saw Mary, the leader of the gang. Lacrista knew the time for threats was over; she sensed that Mary was out for blood.

And she got it. When the fight was over Mary had to be hospitalized and needed stitches to close her wounds.

Lacrista had to fight many times after that. A strong, athletic girl, empowered by the strength of her convictions, Lacrista won each time, and eventually the gangs left her alone.

Lacrista's story, reported by Dirk Johnson in *The New York Times,* is a symbol of hope. Of course, taking on drug dealers in hand-to-hand combat isn't always the solution. But Lacrista embodies the values, the moral strength, and the conviction we need in the fight against drugs.

The Media The Partnership for a Drug-Free America has organized the donation of creative services, airtime, and ad space for a remarkable series of anti-drug advertising messages. Using the same strategies that work to sell goods and services, the Partnership strives to reduce demand by *unselling* drugs. To help reduce the number of first-time drug users, The Partnership first researched this market, then devised prevention messages for specific target audiences. Additional research is conducted annually to see if their messages produced changes in attitude and behavior, and refinements are made accordingly. For example, one radio ad features a pulsing beat and some tough words from rap musicians who snap: "Don't believe the drug man's hype!" Partnership advertising messages are targeted at specific audiences, such as parents, Hispanics, African Americans, and health-care professionals. The dollar value of Partnership's effort amounts to approximately $365 million in donated time and space a year. The value in terms of health and lives saved is incalculable.

Other groups also help spread the word about drugs. The United Way, The Advertising Council, dairy companies, supermarkets, and many other organizations are broadcasting antidrug messages on buses, television public service announcements, milk cartons, and grocery bags. Every little bit helps.

Government I'm proud to have been one of the advisers who consulted with William Bennett and presented the "drug czar's" new aggressive antidrug plan to President Bush and his Cabinet. I am encouraged by the way the government has responded to the issue of drug abuse. Even more, I am pleased that it has backed up its commitment with funds not just for law enforcement and interdiction, but with new funds for treatment, prevention, and education as well. It is a good first step.

Having a strong, coordinated policy at the national level reinforces local and grass-roots efforts. Many states, including the state of New Jersey, have enacted tough new antidrug laws, laws that include such measures as stricter punishments, confiscation of property, and mandatory sentences. Local police departments have made enforcement of drug policies their number one priority. We'll take a closer look at some of these developments in Chapter Twelve.

In short, drugs are falling out of favor. We still have far to go, but today, even in the worst neighborhoods, many kids now have the guts to say no to drugs. Students are catching on to the risks involved. The nation as a whole has seen the need for a change, and is working hard to bring it about.

The Drug Strategy for the 1990s

The way we effect change in America is person to person. As any politician knows, speaking before large crowds is fine, but the way to get votes is to meet people one-on-one, talk about their concerns, and listen to their suggestions. My strategy is similar: We must get the message to each schoolchild, every mother and father, each local community, every employer and employee. We must learn from each other the facts about the nature of drug abuse, its causes and effects, and involve everybody in working out solutions. We must share our information—successes and failures—so that everyone has access to the sharpest and most powerful tools possible in order to continue chipping away at this problem.

Educate and Prevent Education is the single most powerful weapon we wield. As Thomas Jefferson observed, "Enlighten the people generally, and tyranny and oppression of body and mind will vanish like evil spirits at the dawn of day."

We spend millions of dollars educating smokers on the dangers of their habit—education that has worked. We have done an incredible job educating ourselves on the need for healthy diets and exercise. Now we need to apply that energy to teaching people about the dangers of drugs.

The key, though, is to educate people *to prevent them from beginning drug use or to teach them why they should stop.* Without a doubt, prevention is the most humane and cost-effective strategy we can adopt.

Education for prevention actually begins before a child is even conceived. Would-be parents need to know the terrible price their baby will pay if they use drugs and then have a child. Drugs can damage eggs or sperm cells; that damage can in turn affect the ability of the fetus to grow. Mothers must learn that drugs pass through the placenta and are absorbed by the growing baby. Tragically, thousands of babies are born each year *already addicted to cocaine and other drugs.* Drug-using parents must be taught to change their ways if they want happy, thriving children.

After the birth of their child, parents continue to be our most important allies in the drug wars. The values they teach and the loving discipline they administer contribute to a child's sense of self-esteem—an essential weapon if the child is to resist pressure to use drugs in the future.

I believe that every school in the country should implement a compulsive antidrug program as part of their curriculum, and that such programs should begin the first day the child walks into the school. Ultimately, the goal of education is to prevent people from initiating the use of drugs in the first place. As President Bush's Secretary of Education, Lauro F. Cavazos, has stated: "Helping young people to say 'no' to that first drink or that first joint is easier than treating addictions and rebuilding trust in families shattered by drugs."

Learning to say no is crucial because the younger the age at which children begin using any drugs, including alcohol and tobacco, the sooner they will experiment with the "harder stuff." A kid who begins using tobacco learns how to ingest chemicals by smoking. Once he has passed through that threshold, it's much easier for him to make the decision to smoke dope or crack cocaine. For this reason, alcohol, tobacco, and marijuana are considered "gateway" drugs. By the same token, people who do not smoke marijuana rarely move on to try other drugs. Thus, to prevent cocaine use, we need to make a strong case against marijuana; to prevent marijuana use, we need to emphasize the hazards of cigarettes and alcohol.

One educational technique that we know does *not* work is

the passive approach, whereby teachers present the bare facts of drug use without offering a moral perspective. Such methods serve merely to stimulate youngsters' curiosity about drugs, and nothing to steer them toward making the right choice, or give them the tools to actually say no when confronted. I advocate *education for prevention*—teaching the facts *and* taking an active stance against drugs.

Change Social Attitudes Change needs direction from the top. Carlton Turner, President Reagan's drug advisor, Ian MacDonald, M.D., pediatrician and drug prevention advocate, and Nancy Reagan were instrumental in creating a new, anti-drug era. The White House Conference for a Drug Free America, commissioned by Ronald Reagan, said in its Final Report:

> When the average American condemns illegal drug use by their children, their neighbors, themselves; when we all refuse to buy products that sponsor magazines, movies, and television programs glamorizing drugs; when we no longer name as heroes sports figures or entertainers who use drugs—we will all know we are serious about ending the use of illegal drugs in America.

As I've shown, we've come a long way in reducing social tolerance for drug use. Still, there's much work to be done.

Tests for Drugs In their treaty negotiations, the superpowers operate under a simple rule of thumb: "Trust—but verify." The same maxim applies in the war on drugs. Urine drug testing, whether as part of a medical exam or as a requirement for employment, is perhaps the most effective form of prevention available.

As a drug specialist, I know that testing is absolutely essential if treatment is to work. My patients know that I trust them to stay off drugs, but that I intend to verify whether they have been able to keep their word. The purpose of testing is not to blame or criticize. But if I am to help them achieve their goal of becoming drug-free, I need to know if they are lying to me or themselves, or if they are unable to keep away from drugs. Without that knowledge I am crippled in my efforts to find the right form of treatment and help free them from their drug prison.

I advocate drug testing as a strategy at just about every level, from the routine physical exam to the workplace. In some cases, parents should even consider having their children tested periodically. An invasion of privacy? No—a strong signal of parental love and concern that dramatizes the seriousness with which parents regard drug use. An unexpected positive test can help the family act before formal treatment is necessary.

The question of whether or not urine tests are themselves an invasion of privacy may soon become a moot point. In the very near future, drug tests using strands of hair may replace other forms of testing. A drug-user's hair contains traces of illegal drugs in amounts that reveal the length and extent of a person's drug use.

Provide Quality Treatment Any plan for winning the drug war must include wide access to drug treatment programs. A wide range of treatment programs, from outpatient evening programs to long-term residential programs should be available in every community. We must also keep working to improve the quality and effectiveness of care.

Today we know that some people are biologically predisposed to addiction, and that their cultural environment can trigger a plunge into a chemical hell. Of equal importance, we know how to intervene to block those triggers. We also realize that the value of strong emotional support provided by groups such as Alcoholics Anonymous and other "Twelve Step" programs is incalculable. We must be sure to provide a range of treatment options for anyone who needs it.

This range of treatment options should be tailored to the individual addict. In the past, all addicts—especially alcoholics—were treated alike. Today we realize that the treatment needs of a 40-year-old executive are far different than what a 17-year-old unemployed high school dropout requires. My colleague Herbert D. Kleber, M.D. agrees, saying recently that these young unemployed users need "not rehabilitation but habilitation. They may need a range of social services, counseling, and job training in order to have a productive life." Other, more-publicized treatment proposals, such as Treatment on Demand may be more symbolic than important in matching treatment to patient. In fact one study of patients who were treated for their drug abuse within 7 days of their first appointment did not fare any better in treatment than those who waited longer.

Finally, there is one essential stratagem that cannot be overlooked . . .

Target a New War Against Drugs in Our Cities While the vast majority of Americans have heard and heeded the antidrug message, significant segments of our society have not. In the past, illicit drug use has followed a "first in/first out" pattern. For example, in recent years the wealthiest were the first to experiment with cocaine, the first to be devastated by it, and the first to seek treatment.

Unfortunately our poorest classes currently do not have the resources necessary to withstand or rebound from the drug onslaught. Many are now daily or continuous users, a group for whom otherwise powerful persuasive techniques such as media messages and deterrents such as job jeopardy have little effect. Hence, addiction and new drug use among the poorest citizens continue to be problems today—especially in our inner cities where black and hispanic children are virtually surrounded by drug use. Surveys conducted for the Partnership for a Drug-Free America by the Gordon S. Black Corporation (GSBC) have found that the antidrug attitudes of black and hispanic teenagers do not match those of white teenagers. For example, when asked if they agreed either "strongly" or "moderately" with the statement "Cocaine is not harmful if used only occasionally," only 11 percent of white teenagers answered yes, compared to 21 percent of black and 22 percent of hispanic teens.

Compounding these differences in attitude is the greater exposure of black children to drugs. A GSBC survey found that 27 percent of black children aged nine to 12 years have been approached to buy or use drugs, compared to only 13 percent of white children. Black and hispanic children are asked to try drugs at an earlier age and with greater frequency. Repeatedly, they are put in the dangerous position of having to say no to drugs.

Clearly, a new tactic in the drug war is necessary, one that emphasizes reducing drug use in the city through a broad-based approach that—in addition to continuing existing educational efforts—includes:

- a targeted effort to identify and treat addicts.
- greater emphasis on maternal infant care, including residential centers where pregnant women can live and receive optimal prenatal care, and educational and emotional group support.
- additional police patrols in drug-infested sections of cities to minimize the exposure of children and other innocent citizens to drugs, drug sellers, and drug-related crime, while helping innocent citizens to regain control of their streets.
- the creation of a civil rights commission to study how drugs have preferentially blighted black and hispanic Americans and to suggest means of legally and effectively curing this problem.
- increase basic research and discover an emergency antidote for cocaine overdose and toxicity.
- a pilot project for an urban public-works job corps where full-time work is dependent upon attending self-help meetings and passing drug tests.
- a pilot project using the kibbutz or commune as a model for a long-term treatment program for families.
- support for grass-root programs that work, such as the East Tenth Street Block Association in New York City, whose work with police and city government officials has resulted in police barricades that shut down the street during peak drug-buying times.

With a newly targeted program, America's overall victories in the war against drugs can be duplicated in our cities.

Difficult? Yes. But I think by the time you finish this book you'll agree that we've made tremendous strides against drugs, and that there is strong reason for hope.

And that is very good news indeed.

CHAPTER TWO

How Drugs Became America's Number One Problem

"Turn On, Tune In, Drop Out."

The phrase that symbolized the sixties almost destroyed a generation.

Just look at what this slogan promised: Use drugs and you can be one of us—the inner circle of those who *really* know what's going on. Use drugs and you'll leave behind the evils of the establishment that created the Vietnam War, pollution, racism, the threat of nuclear war, and poverty. Use drugs and together we can find Nirvana—a utopia in our heads and in our lives. Use drugs and even "strawberry fields" can last "forever." No wonder millions were seduced by this message.

In the mid-1960s, drug use exploded at a time when:

- America was tormented by an unpopular war;
- Rachel Carson's *Silent Spring* warned against widespread ecological disaster;
- lives were being lost in the battle for civil rights;
- a popular American president had just been assassinated;
- popular music and rock stars made fighting the establishment "in."
- Books and movies like *Dr. Strangelove* made fun of the

military while bringing our fears of nuclear destruction into the open.

The world was seemingly on the "eve of destruction" and something—anything—was necessary to stop the slide. We were all looking for answers. The slogan "If you're not part of the solution, you're part of the problem" said it all.

For many, drugs became *the* answer. If everybody just got high, there wouldn't be any war—only love. When you were high, the problems of the world either didn't matter, or they didn't seem so bad. That's what people used to think. In that era, drugs became so intertwined with "relevant" issues that they became a "litmus test"—use drugs and you were one of "us." Refuse to use drugs and you were one of them—the establishment responsible for Vietnam, for poverty, and for pollution.

But why did drug use persist, even flourish, in the decades following 1969—long after the Nehru jackets, black-light posters, lava lights, and liberal college students had disappeared?

This question is difficult to answer, and yet it is one that every individual—especially those veterans of the "Days of Rage"—must ask themselves.

It's not that the ideals of the sixties should be dismissed; rather they should be seen in the proper light, divested of their illusory association with drugs. The fight for civil rights should never be used to defend a person's "right" to take drugs; the road to personal freedom isn't lined by coke; a clean environment means a lifestyle free from all harmful chemicals, including THC.

Did the people who took drugs in the 1960s really believe that drugs could change the world? No, not really. What they believed—or thought they believed—was an illusion, one as old as cocaine itself. Illusion and drugs go hand-in-hand.

But the 1980s have shown us that the 1960s did not hold a monopoly upon illusions and drugs. The following history of drug use clearly indicates how drugs and illusions have conspired to create a legacy of false promises, counterfeit hopes, and ruined lives.

Drug Abuse: A History of Illusion

• In 1850, cannabis appeared in the *U.S. Pharmacopeia* and numerous pharmaceutical firms touted it as a natural herbal cure.

• In the late 1850s, a new, coca-containing elixir called Vin Mariani (after its creator, chemist Angelo Mariani) debuted as a "cure-all," endorsed by such respected authorities as Thomas Edison and Pope Leo XIII.

• In 1884, Sigmund Freud recommended cocaine as a cure for morphine addiction, for digestive disorders, and to treat asthma.

• In 1885, a new "health drink" similar to Vin Mariani and sold in drugstores as Coca-Cola came on the scene.

• Also in 1885, the Parke-Davis Pharmaceutical company called cocaine potentially "the most important therapeutic discovery of the age."

Before 1906, all kinds of nostrums and tonics were available to cure everything from dropsy to diarrhea. Because no regulations existed as to what could or could not be included in these medicines, just about anything went. These so-called "patent medicines" might contain high amounts of alcohol, morphine, heroin, cocaine—or even combinations of these ingredients. They often did nothing to cure what ailed you, but they might get you so high you forgot you were sick! Manufacturers were under no compulsion to list their products' ingredients, although they loved to identify certain critical elements. It is from this era that we get our term "snake oil," which today means a worthless promise of a cure-all.

Before long, reality punctured the illusion of drugs. In 1887, in his paper "Craving For and Fear of Cocaine" Freud called the drug "a far more dangerous enemy to health than morphine." Soon, reports of cocaine addiction flooded the medical journals. Then the first backlash against cocaine began:

• In 1901, the American Pharmacological Association condemned cocaine.

• In 1906, the Pure Food and Drug Act severely limited the use of cocaine in medications and elixirs. The so-called medical usages of cocaine, as well as the drugstore cocaine-based elixirs, disappeared within a very short time.

After decades of what amounted to a massive social experiment with drugs, aided by an unregulated pharmaceutical industry and abetted by unsuspecting physicians, the problem of snake-oil cures and unregulated drug use became enormous. In 1914, the federal government passed the Harrison Narcotic Act to regulate the ways in which physicians could dispense drugs. That legislation helped keep drugs out of the hands of many people, but forced those who were already addicted to become criminals in order to feed their habits.

Prohibition: Success or Failure?

A few years later our society targeted alcohol, also produced by an unregulated industry, as the next drug-based vice that needed control. In 1920, the Eighteenth Amendment, known as the Prohibition Amendment, was ratified.

Some social critics claim that Prohibition was a colossal failure. It didn't stop drinking, they say; all it did was turn the business of making and selling alcoholic beverages over to bootleggers and criminals.

But in many ways, Prohibition succeeded. For example, Prohibition:

• reduced drinking by one-third;

• produced a 64 percent drop in deaths from cirrhosis;

• resulted in a 53 percent decline in admissions to mental hospitals.

Had the prohibition laws been tougher and more aggressively enforced, the benefits to society would have been even greater. We need to keep this important fact in mind as the debate over legalizing drugs heats up.

From Prohibition to the Present

Still trying to control the chemical state of the union, Congress passed the Marijuana Tax Act in 1937, thus placing marijuana on the growing list of forbidden substances.

For decades, however, the strongest force in controlling drug use was social censure. Possibly as a result of attitudes nourished during the Prohibition era, people began to look at excessive drinking as a sign of moral weakness or failure. Though movies portrayed drug addicts as obvious junkies, losers, and misfits, people barely acknowledged the fact that thousands of otherwise normal citizens abused drugs and alcohol and managed to live seemingly normal lives. Heroin became the primary drug of abuse. But since heroin users lived mainly in urban ghettos, they seldom came into contact with the mainstream of society and could be conveniently ignored.

The substance abuse picture changed after World War II. One major factor in this change was the arrival in the 1950s of new types of powerful medications with the ability to alter mood. Physicians could now treat such common problems as anxiety and depression at the drop of a pill. The practice of psychiatry changed forever. Now, patients who had problems coping with life and who formerly subjected themselves to years of psychoanalysis found their spirits lifting after mere weeks of treatment with antidepressant medications. Ironically, some of the same people who saw heroin addicts as pathetic losers became hooked on tranquilizers and other mood-altering prescription drugs that were many times more potent than heroin. By the early 1960s, relief for virtually any type of problem was just a pill away.

Small wonder, then, that other mind-changing chemicals, new and otherwise, appeared and took hold. Marijuana came into its own as the drug of choice of a new generation. Young people experimented with LSD and other hallucinogens, as a recreational activity, as part of a spiritual quest, and as a way of thumbing their noses at society. While never legal, use of these chemicals was more widely tolerated than ever before.

The market for drugs grew so large during this time that a huge worldwide network of growers, manufacturers, and distributors sprang up. Anyone with access to some basic lab equipment, a few easily obtained raw materials, and a working knowledge of chemistry could whip up a batch of LSD, cocaine, or other black market items such as amphetamines or barbiturates. In large measure, the existence of this sophisticated and profitable underground industry led to the drug abuse epidemic we see today.

Acceptance led to accessibility. Users no longer had to haunt the alleyways of the city; drugs changed hands on campuses, in high schools, and in the workplace. Marijuana didn't have to be imported. Entrepreneurs grew patches of the weed in their backyards, in specially lighted closets, in isolated rural areas, even on federal property within national parks. Today marijuana is still the largest cash crop in several American states.

Tolerance to alcohol increased as well. Many states lowered the drinking age to 18, the same age at which people could vote or join the army.

If the sixties are remembered as the era of widespread experimentation with drugs, the seventies will be remembered as the decade in which drug use became an epidemic. Cocaine, especially, emerged as a glamour drug, the "champagne of pharmaceuticals," used by the glitterati, the high rollers, athletes, movie stars, and rock stars. As usual, Joe and Jane Everyperson felt compelled to emulate the examples of these glamorous, high-profile trendsetters.

Demand was high; so was supply. For every 100 pounds of illegal drugs headed for America, 90 pounds made it through. The stuff was so abundant that prices plummeted. Practically anyone could afford drugs. Cocaine cost $75 or less per gram; an ounce of pot went for perhaps $40.

With cheap abundant drugs available everywhere, the party shifted into high gear. Snorting coke was still popular, but the new kick was to use a smokable form of cocaine called freebase.

Some people mixed cocaine with heroin in a combination called a "speedball." The comedian John Belushi liked this formula. It killed him.

So-called "experts" made headlines by claiming that they used cocaine and that they knew—ipso facto—that cocaine was perfectly safe—as safe as chicken soup. Meanwhile warnings that cocaine was very dangerous went unheeded, even when laboratories showed that animals preferred cocaine over food, sex, or sleep—the only thing that could interrupt their drug use was death!—and even when reports proved that "pure" cocaine contained large amounts of other substances. Users who devoted every waking minute to obtaining and snorting coke scoffed at the notion that the drug was addictive. To back up their claim, they pointed to interviews with authorities who said coke use was merely a compulsive act, like drinking coffee or eating potato chips.

As a doctor who had to treat these substance abusers, such remarks make me grind my teeth.

Out of concern for this growing epidemic, I founded the 24-hour, national, 800-COCAINE telephone helpline in the spring of 1983; we took our very first phone call on May 6, 1983—before virtually any other cocaine program had started. The goal was to provide a resource for users who needed facts, guidance, and treatment. I predicted we might get a few dozen calls a day. The day we opened the switchboard I appeared on the *Today* show to announce the number. By the time I drove back to my office in New Jersey, about 30 miles away, the helpline had been flooded—nearly a hundred calls. And each hour, as *Today* was broadcast in different time zones across the country, even more calls poured in. I couldn't stop answering the phone. "Am I addicted?" and "Is treatment possible?" were the most common questions. The stories our callers told us confirmed what I had seen with my own eyes, what the labs had reported, and what the experts had been blind to: that cocaine is dangerous. Use of cocaine builds up tolerance, which leads to dependency and ultimately to addiction. Once you are addicted, it is extremely hard to stop.

Unless disaster does the stopping for you.

Within a few years 800-COCAINE had logged over one million calls for help—roughly 1,500 a day. The calls gave my colleagues Don Sweeney, Arnold Washton, Bill Annitto, Carter Pottash, and Jim Cocores—who looked at the surveys and talked to callers during the first years—an instant understanding of what was happening in the country and provided a startling profile of modern-day cocaine users. While many callers were loved ones of users, the typical callers were average, middle class, well-educated, well-paid people who used the drug almost daily, and whose family lives and careers were beginning to fall apart because of their devotion to cocaine.

In the mid-1980s two important developments changed the picture of cocaine use in America. The first was the sudden, shocking death of several promising young athletes due to cocaine use. One story had particular impact—that of basketball player Len Bias. After a brilliant college career, Bias was on the verge of professional stardom and financial success when he used cocaine apparently for the first time. It was also the last thing he did. This young, perfectly healthy man collapsed and was rushed, still alive, to a hospital. The doctors examined him but could do nothing for him. *There is no treatment for cocaine overdose.* The doctors tried but were helpless as cocaine snuffed out his life.

Soon another prominent athlete, Don Rodgers, a star defensive back for the Cleveland Browns, also died from a cocaine overdose. Bias and Rodgers did not die completely in vain: their tragedies prompted many people—famous athletes, celebrities, and noncelebrities alike—to admit that they had a drug problem and to seek treatment. Their deaths crushed the myth that occasional use or cocaine snorting was safe.

Before the mid-1980s, many experts believed that coke's high price would limit its popularity among adolescents. Others smugly reported adolescents would only drink or smoke their drugs.

Well, high prices were soon no longer a problem. Along came crack cocaine, the second key development in the cocaine picture. Distributed in inexpensive amounts and very powerful, this insidious smokable form of coke gives users an intensely pleasurable rush of euphoria within seconds of lighting the pipe. Because a dose of crack costs as little as $3 and is smokeable, it is available to just about anybody—even a schoolkid with lunch money in his pocket. As we'll see in Chapter Seven, the crack high is so intense that it stimulates users to repeat the dose, leading quickly to addiction and thus ensuring dealers of a steady supply of customers.

"Oh, don't worry," some experts said calmly. "Crack is merely a phenomenon of the urban ghetto. It'll never catch on outside of New York or Florida or California. Besides, cocaine isn't *really* addictive—not in a physical sense. It's only psychologically addicting. People just *think* they're hooked."

Guess again. Linda Semlitz, Arnold Washton, and the staff at 800-COCAINE profiled the adolescent user and tracked the spread of adolescent drug use. Crack is showing up in every big city, a lot of middle-sized cities, and even in small towns and rural areas. And it is most definitely addicting—sometimes instantly so. The calls now flooding the 800-COCAINE switchboard confirm that crack is the single most significant event in the drug history of this nation since the psychedelic sixties.

One constant in this history has been people's willful blindness to the dangers of drugs. The American attitude seems to be that all drugs are innocent—that is, harmless—until proven guilty. "Look at the pot smokers of decades past," people say. "They were zonked on dope for years, but they grew up to be typical middle class individuals, with families, homes, and careers. They turned out okay. Their kids have the right number of fingers and toes. Some former users even became Congressmen. By extension, then, *all* drugs must be okay."

I often hear such misguided, misinformed rationalizations, especially from younger patients—the very people most vulnerable to drugs. It's ironic that as a society we demand that our pharmaceutical companies spend years and millions of dollars testing their products for safety and efficacy before we allow them on the market. But we'll swallow huge quantities of unlabeled and untested pills, from unknown makers, that are sold to us in dark alleys by perfect strangers and assume these products are totally harmless.

A parallel attitude is that of *denial.* Users deny they have a problem—"I can quit anytime," they say, as they scramble frantically to get money to buy another dose. "I control drugs, they don't control me," they claim, as their brains and bodies rot under the onslaught of chemical intoxication. But even nonusers tend to deny that the problem exists. "My kid's not on drugs," a parent says. "We've eliminated drug use in our fair city," claims the mayoral candidate running for reelection. "Our school is drug-free," boasts the principal. None of these people will acknowledge that the problem is rampant. To do so would mean admitting that they aren't doing their jobs very well.

Belief in such myths has led directly to the drug mess we're in today. That's the trouble with having an attitude of tolerance: It carries over from one drug to another, and causes users of one chemical to become more likely to try another, more dangerous one.

In summary, for more than two decades now our society has experimented with drugs on an enormous scale, under the false assumption that they are safe. In a sense, we have field-tested these drugs on millions of people. Only now, with incontestable data at hand, can we look at the results of this "field test" and state our conclusions with certainty: Drugs are dangerous, addictive, and deadly.

Factors that Lead to Drug Use

I remember the 1982 comment of my overworked colleague Don Sweeney, M.D., the Fair Oaks clinical director, as we struggled to keep up with the growing numbers of drug users: "You know, the guys on Madison Avenue can make us recoil in horror at the thought of 'ring around the collar,' bad breath, and dandruff flakes. They can even make us buy toilet paper that's 'squeezably soft.' Why can't they make people realize that cocaine isn't sexy, that it makes your nose bleed, that it can kill you?" At that time cocaine was being "marketed" as an elite, hip, power drug. We didn't understand that advertising could "unsell" a product.

Well, a few years ago, Dr. Sweeney got his wish. In 1986, some of the country's best advertising, marketing, and media moguls formed the Partnership for a Drug-Free America. Not only has this organization produced some of the most effective antidrug campaigns to date, but it has also sponsored comprehensive surveys—conducted by the Gordon S. Black Corporation (GSBC)—that reflect the attitudes of Americans toward drugs. Each survey provides new insights and new targets for educating users and "unselling" drugs. These surveys, conducted with the same thoroughness normally reserved for dishwater liquid and politicians, have provided invaluable information that has helped shape our most effective antidrug efforts. These surveys also suggest why some children, adolescents, and adults use drugs while others do not. For example, The Partnership surveys found that both *marijuana and cocaine use are already established by age 13*. Consider these 1990 findings:

- Fifteen percent of children nine to 12 years of age have already been approached to buy or use drugs.
- Ten percent of these nine to 12-year-olds say that it's easy to get cocaine and crack.
- Approximately 20 percent of these pre-teens have tried alcohol and cigarettes.

Clearly, exposure to drugs is a major factor in drug use. But *lack of exposure*—to antidrug messages—may also be a major component. These surveys have been very useful in tracking the importance of drug education.

In 1987, before the first wave of the Partnership's advertising and media campaign had begun, the Gordon S. Black Corporation surveyed the attitudes of children, teenagers, and adults in "high media" areas (areas likely to receive a 50 percent greater exposure to the Partnership's advertising campaign). One year later, *after* the Partnership's antidrug campaign had begun, they repeated the survey.

In just one year the results were striking: *In almost every instance,* the antidrug attitudes in 1988 surpassed the attitudes of 1987, with the antidrug attitudes in high media areas consistently beating the low or moderate media areas. The following is just a sampling of the survey's findings:

- Children, teens, and adults in high media areas have become more antidrug.
- Children in high media areas are talking about drugs more.
- More teens in high media areas disagree with prodrug statements.
- Parents in high media areas are taking more action against drugs.

Perhaps most important, the 1988 survey found that *"among the college students, where attitudinal changes appear the greatest, there are statistically significant declines in cocaine consumption, primarily among the 'occasional user.'"*

Subsequent surveys conducted in 1989 and 1990 proved that the 1988 survey was not a one-year fluke. In fact, a 1990 Partnership survey found that:

- from 1987 to 1990, the number of teens using cocaine dropped from 11 to 6 percent.
- the number of teens using marijuana decreased from 29 percent in 1987 to 21 percent in 1990.

Furthermore, preliminary results from a study of high schools in Kansas City—conducted by the National Institute of Drug Abuse—indicate the success of drug abuse prevention programs. This study has found that only 1.6 percent of students who participated in the drug abuse prevention program had used drugs within the last 30 days, compared to 3.7 percent for students who had not participated in the program.

Dual Diagnosis: The Double Trouble of Substance Abuse and Psychiatric Disorders After years of struggling to establish addiction as a separate disease, we are just now beginning to understand the many factors that can complicate its detection and treatment. Foremost among these factors is dual diagnosis. Just as hypertension and kidney disease are often found together, addiction and psychiatric disorders such as depression and anxiety frequently coexist. Recent large-scale studies from the National Institute of Mental Health have found that 18 percent of people with a history of depression and 41 percent who had suffered from manic depression also had abused drugs. Other studies of patients being treated for alcoholism have found that 50 percent suffered from anxiety and panic disorders. Cocaine abusers show a co-existing mental illness rate that exceeds 76 percent! This association has resulted in researchers who were primarily concerned with psychiatric subjects becoming involved in drug-abuse research. One research pioneer, Fred Goodwin, chief of the Alcohol, Drug Abuse and Mental Health Administration (ADAMHA) is currently working with some of the best minds to unravel a number of drug-abuse puzzles.

Why is there such an amazing affinity between addiction and psychiatric disorders? Anyone who has ever suffered from depression or anxiety disorders will tell you how alluring even the faintest promise of relief from their unhappiness can be. Alcohol, cocaine, or marijuana offer false hopes of lifting the person's torment. In the short run, this form of self-medication may work, but over time the person's suffering intensifies and the depression or anxiety returns with even greater vengeance.

In addition to anxiety and depression, other problems such as learning disabilities and Attention Deficit Hyperactivity Disorder may contribute to substance abuse. Often these conditions lead to feelings of hopelessness, ignorance, inadequacy, and low self-esteem. While these feelings can disrupt anyone's life, they are especially tough on teens.

For teenagers with low self-esteem, drugs and alcohol can help fill the void and overcome their sense of hopelessness. In fact, among the factors that lead kids to experiment with drugs and alcohol, lack of self-esteem ranks number one. The problem is that once these teens learn the drug "solution" to their problems, they are more likely to continue resorting to that solution throughout their lives, whenever stress or unhappiness arises.

High-potency drugs Recently, during a family therapy session with a 15-year-old named Tamara and her parents, we focused on the ways that attitudes at home were contributing to her current drug abuse problem—daily use of marijuana and alcohol, and frequent cocaine use.

"What's so bad about smoking pot?" Tamara's father Rhys asked. "I smoked it when I was a kid. So did my wife. We don't think we were harmed by it."

"Did you ever smoke 30 joints at once?" I asked.

"God, no," he answered.

"I want you to understand something," I said. "The marijuana your daughter is buying on the street today could be as much as *30 times as powerful* as the pot you smoked in college."

As Rhys stared at me in disbelief, I explained: THC is the active ingredient in marijuana, the thing that makes you high. A typical joint from, say, 1970 might have contained one-half to one percent THC—a dose of about 10 milligrams. The stuff we analyze in our labs today, though, can have as much as 150 milligrams of THC—15 percent by weight. Reports from California indicate that some pot can contain even higher amounts—up to 20 percent. If it's laced with hashish oil, as some of the pot today is, you can pretty much double those figures. I told Rhys his daughter may be getting a more intense high from one joint than if she smoked dozens of the ones he used to roll.

Perhaps because we doctors have not been very effective in spreading the word, many people like Rhys and his family fail to realize that drugs today are much more potent than they were just a few years ago. Worse, at such high doses, marijuana has serious long-term effects. Studies show that in as little as eleven days' time, a daily dose of 180 milligrams of THC—a joint or two—produces a defined withdrawal syndrome. Symptoms include insomnia, nausea, muscle aches, restlessness, and irritability. In fact, this new high-potency pot—the product of sophisticated growing techniques and genetic selection—is actually just as addictive as cocaine or hashish. This greater intoxicating power means that everything we thought we knew about the risks and consequences of marijuana is now obsolete.

Thus, people who say "pot is safe" are not talking about a product that has been tested by the Food and Drug Administration. Where marijuana supporters are concerned, the typical burden of proof for a drug's safety is reversed; i.e. in their minds drugs are safe until proven dangerous.

Cocaine, too, is more powerful than before. Much of its potency depends on the route of administration. The effect of smoking crack can be ten times as strong as snorting cocaine powder. Smoking cocaine sends the fumes into the lungs, a highly efficient biological system designed to allow molecules (oxygen, of course, but cocaine as well) to be absorbed into the bloodstream. Once absorbed, nearly the entire dose of cocaine circulates quickly to the brain. Sniffing cocaine, however, prevents much of the dose from entering the bloodstream. The nose acts as a terrific filter for impurities—that's its job, after all. The part of the dose that does get absorbed takes much longer to make its way to the brain.

Before 1985, our 800-COCAINE surveys showed that a typical cocaine addiction took nearly four and a half years to develop. After the advent of crack, however, addiction could take hold within a few months—even weeks. Part of the good news about drugs is that the number of cocaine users is dropping. The downside, though, is that those who still use coke do so more often—once a week or more. There are fewer users, but their rate of use is higher and their addiction stronger.

Drug Marketing Strategies Drug use offered the user access to a sub-culture, a peer group with its own rituals, common experience, language, music, and ethics. Drug dealers—astute observers of human behavior that they are—exploit the user's mentality. They discern their customers' weak points and focus their efforts there. They market their wares like any other respectable American manufacturer. Dealers offer free samples, discount prices, commissions, and other incentives to their top salesmen. They advertise (by word of mouth, mostly), make exaggerated claims, and downplay the risks. One enterprising crack salesman even offered his steady clients "two-for-one" specials on Sundays! As he told a reporter for *Time* magazine,

"I always believe in treating my customer good." Worse, such dealers often sell more than one type of drug. They are, in fact, walking drugstores. A kid who knows a good source for, say, marijuana is highly likely to be exposed to other drugs as well. The first sample is usually free; later doses, however, will cost dearly. The cocaine epidemic is a tragic example of how drugs are sold to millions—using drugs becomes symbolic of affluence, an elite class with ties to celebrity endorsements.

Family Attitudes As we saw with Tamara's family, parental attitudes do make a difference—not just about illicit drugs but about alcohol, cigarettes, and even caffeine. We know, too, that having a sibling who uses drugs is one of the largest factors in a young person's decision to try them. In Chapter 16 we'll see how a complete treatment program for drug abuse involves correcting the faulty assumptions, beliefs, and behaviors of everyone in the home, not just the "patient of record."

What Have We Done to Stop Drug Use?

It's a recurring theme of the history of drugs in this country: Our attitudes of tolerance and acceptance have led to more widespread use. We also know the psychological and social risk factors that contribute to the choice to experiment with drugs. Given those facts, the question arises: Wasn't anybody doing anything to curb drug use?

Yes and no. Yes, of course, steps were taken; no, some of them didn't do as much as we hoped.

In the past those who wanted to put an end to drugs tended to focus their energies on *interdiction*—on blocking the flow of drugs before they reach the consumer. This might mean anything from defoliating marijuana or coca fields to clamping down on drug dealing in the streets.

In the past decade or so, the federal government tripled the amount of money spent on drug law enforcement. As a result, some huge drug caches were seized. The headline writers had a field day: "Multimillion-dollar drug shipment intercepted at sea!" "Tons of pot found in suburban basements!" But these seizures represent just the tip of the iceberg. They helped to keep us from seeing 25-cent crack rocks and 10-dollar grams of cocaine, but as I noted earlier, 90 percent of cocaine headed for this country makes its way across the border. Interdiction has kept the price artificially high and made it difficult for drug criminals to enjoy their money. Asset forfeiture—a policy where a drug dealer's profits are turned over to the government—has put added teeth into police efforts.

Interdiction has caused rises in the street prices of drugs, with a corresponding drop in use. But is it our most effective weapon against drugs today? As one Washington analyst stated, busting pushers "is like trying to put General Motors out of business by knocking off used-car dealers." And trying to get other nations to cooperate by squashing powerful and ruthless drug lords and destroying their drug-producing plants—for some countries, their largest source of income—is notoriously difficult. For that matter, even if every coca leaf on earth were suddenly destroyed, drug entrepreneurs could make artificial cocaine in basement labs using a few easily obtainable raw materials.

Jack Lawn, head of the Drug Enforcement Administration under President Reagan, realized the limitations of interdiction and was instrumental in the new emphasis on demand reduction. But would demand reduction really work? Here again, the answer is yes and no. We *can* reduce demand—if we do it right. But over the past few years, we've gone about the job in ways that sometimes have been ineffective.

For a time people believed we could prevent drug abuse by addressing the personal factors—attitudes, beliefs, and values—that influence the decision to try drugs. Other programs tried simply to distract young people by offering alternative activities, such as sports or recreational programs. The hope was to pull the kid out of his boredom, remove him from peer pressure to try drugs, and give him a sense of belonging. These approaches did work for some teens, but they were not the most effective antidrug strategies.

In recent years the trend has shifted to a direction I have advocated all along: Education For Prevention. But just teaching the facts isn't enough. Telling a kid that there's a drug out there that within ten seconds will give him so much pleasure he may experience a feeling equal to sexual orgasm is only going to pique his curiosity. In the name of objectivity, past antidrug campaigns failed to accurately stress the essential fact: Drugs are dangerous. Today, antidrug education must include that message—the most important fact of all.

But there's another crucial aspect to education that we often neglect. We must also teach young people how to develop the psychological and social skills they need to resist peer pressure. In other words, yes, we must get the message across—say no to drugs—but we also must make sure kids know *how* to say no. Efforts along these lines include role-playing, group discussions, and other techniques that enable kids to rehearse their responses to threatening situations.

In the past we've taught kids to "yell and tell" if someone tried to molest them; we've told them to "drop and roll" if their clothes catch on fire. Now we have to show them ways to "push back the pushers." More details on this strategy appear in Chapter Twelve.

Lately we've seen encouraging signs of progress. There's still much to be done. Two noted researchers with the National Institute of Drug Abuse, R. M. Battjes and C. L. Jones, have come up with a list of proven prevention techniques, which I want to include here:

- Start early. And I do mean *early.* Grab them as kindergarteners and keep hammering away at each grade level. The age of first drug use is dropping. It's too late to "prevent" a 15-year-old from trying marijuana if she's already smoked it at age 11, as so many do.
- Single-strategy approaches won't cut it. There are too many different kinds of drugs, too many different kinds of users with different reasons for experimenting with substances. If prevention programs have any prayer of succeeding, they have to be targeted for *specific* types of people and *specific* drug-use behavior.

• We have to be aware of the many psychological and psychiatric problems that may lead some people to use drugs. Just saying no won't work for a person with a behavioral disorder, personality problem, or clinical depression.

• Antidrug programs have to know their market. As I mentioned, adolescents love to take risks. That's often what leads to experimentation in the first place. Thus, to be effective, a prevention program must work with that risk-taking impulse and redirect it. Ignoring it, or trying to eliminate it, will ultimately fail.

• Include alcohol and tobacco as targets for prevention. We now know for a fact that use of these substances serves as a gateway to the harder stuff. Prevent a kid from smoking cigarettes and he'll be less likely to try smoking dope.

• Hard facts about drugs are crucial, but those facts have to be communicated by respected and credible authority figures. Better, for example, to train teachers to spread the word than to bring in outside lecturers, people who show up for an hour and are never seen again. Programs must be appropriate to the audience's age, values, and level of development.

In the next chapter I'll explain how progress against substance abuse was thwarted by ignorance and misunderstanding among a group of people who were supposed to be the good guys in the struggle: the medical professionals.

CHAPTER THREE

Medicine, Medical "Experts," and the Drug Epidemic

Let me take you back to the year 1950. I want you to meet a man named Brandon.

Brandon is a soldier, fighting in Korea. And like so many others, he's wounded—a piece of shrapnel is imbedded in his back. He's in pain, but he's alive, and that piece of metal is his ticket home.

Brandon returns to St. Louis, hoping to find a job, to settle down and start a family. Sadly, though, his war injuries keep him in constant pain. Doctors try to help him but fail. As you might expect, he begins to drink, hanging out in bars and nightclubs. And it's at one of these bars that a musician friend introduces Brandon to heroin. It isn't long before he's hooked.

Let's travel forward now to 1958. For some time Brandon has managed to live with his addiction. As long as he gets his daily fix, he can continue on somewhat normally. But lately he's become fed up with his life. He senses that time is passing, and he is no closer to realizing his dreams. He hates himself for being a slave to a drug and suffers from feelings of guilt and depression. He wants to make a clean start, to become a new man—or rather, the "old" man he was before his addiction took over. As the phrase goes, he wants to get rid of the monkey on his back.

So off he goes in search of treatment. Remember, though, this is 1958—the dark ages, as far as medical help for addiction goes. He sees a doctor at the local VA hospital. When the doctor hears about Brandon's heroin habit, he says, barely hiding his contempt: "You don't need a physician. Drug addiction is a mental problem. You need a psychiatrist."

Brandon makes an appointment with the VA's psychiatrist. During the first session he learns his drug use is an antisocial act, a form of psychopathic behavior. Brandon gets the sense that he, the former war hero, is not only a criminal but crazy to boot. The doctor tells Brandon he must come in twice a week for therapy "so we can get to the bottom of the problem and discover what drives you to act in this self-destructive way."

Years go by as Brandon and his psychiatrist explore his childhood and his relationships with his parents, looking for clues that might explain his behavior. Nothing solid turns up to stop his drug use. The doctor shifts his strategy, dwelling on Brandon's deeds in Korea. Does he feel guilty for fighting in the war? For going home alive while his friends stayed (and died)? Is he depressed because he became just another faceless returning veteran after the war? What is the *symbolic* meaning of his pain?

Meanwhile, no closer to the answers, Brandon continues to be addicted. After nearly four years of fruitless therapy, he quits going.

Let's flash forward to 1962 to a medical debate raging at the time. Some far-sighted physicians have suggested that people like Brandon should not be seen as criminals to be locked up or as psychopaths who need to be analyzed. Nor, for that matter, need they be hospitalized, since except for their drug habit they can function pretty well in society. Instead, these physicians have suggested a plan to treat addicts in outpatient clinics to help them through the stages of withdrawal. Nonsense, the leaders of the American Medical Association declare. They label the idea of ambulatory clinics "inadequate and medically unsound." Case closed. Brandon is still on the streets.

Now, it's 1965. Brandon hears that doctors are experimenting with the use of a synthetic opiate called methadone to help heroin addicts kick their habit. He volunteers to participate in a clinical trial. Methadone replaces the heroin-like high, and although it is addicting, it is less sedating than heroin, and can be taken orally once a day. Brandon finds it easier to live a more normal life while on methadone. The idea, his doctors tell him, is to gradually lessen the methadone doses until it is stopped altogether, at which point, hopefully, he will be free of his addiction. But no other forms of therapy are administered. Brandon has never learned to habilitate—to live and function—on his own. Rehabilitation of someone like Brandon, who never learned to habilitate, is very difficult.

The plan works, sort of. Brandon *is* free of his addiction—to heroin. Now he is addicted to methadone, which he receives free from the clinic.

I wish I could tell you this story has a happy ending. But as we reach 1969, we see Brandon, his body weakened by decades of drug use, succumb to illness. The doctors list the official cause of his death as pneumonia.

The *real* cause: lack of research and medical ignorance.

The Experts

If I could travel through time, I would have snatched Brandon out of the medical dark ages, plunked him down at my hospital, and launched him on therapeutic medications starting with clonidine and followed by naltrexone. These wonder drugs are nonaddicting, nonnarcotic, and could initially free him from his addiction and then prevent a relapse. Time travel is science fiction. The treatment I've just described is science *fact.*

For all their years of training, doctors, unfortunately, are no more immune to stupidity than anyone else. Though it frustrates me to say it, doctors are part of the reason we have a serious drug epidemic in this country. For years many medical professionals ignored addicts and misunderstood the nature of addiction, and thus were unable to recognize that treatment could work!

Consider cocaine. I first researched this drug in the early 1970s. Even that long ago, experiments had already proved decisively that lab animals, given free rein to push a button that delivered a dose of cocaine, would continue to self-administer the drug—shunning food, water, even sex—*until they died.* The reports were published, the data were available to everyone: Cocaine was clearly addictive, and could not be used in any controlled way. Just as there is no such thing as being "a little pregnant," there is no such thing as a "little" cocaine habit.

In the 1970s, we needed our medical experts to lead a public outcry against cocaine, to warn of its addictive dangers, and to help plan effective educational, preventative, and treatment options for the upcoming epidemic.

Sadly, what we *needed* and what we *got* were two very different things. In the late 1970s these "experts" proclaimed cocaine as a cure for stage fright, and heralded its ability to improve performance and fortify the body and mind. These experts even claimed that users who overindulged would not seek to use more of the drug! They ignored the available data from the first cocaine epidemic at the turn of the century.

How many lives were ruined because of this advice?

Even as recently as 1984, I found myself arguing with medical colleagues who still weren't convinced that cocaine was dangerous. I felt like bashing my head against the wall when some of these colleagues appeared on national TV and in newspapers declaring that cocaine was being villified by medical alarmists.

These same media mavens loved to claim that cocaine was not addictive. No? What about the *Newsweek* report of a wealthy real estate wizard who sold off his skyscraper, one floor at a time, to support his coke habit, until he literally and figuratively reached the ground floor? I felt ashamed that a newsmagazine had a better handle on the truth about cocaine than many of my fellow physicians.

As I'm sure you've noticed, I think we have too many experts and too little expertise. I could forgive Brandon's doctor for not knowing about clonidine or naltrexone; their new uses hadn't been invented in his time. I could even forgive his analyst for considering addiction a form of psychopathology rather than a physical illness; he was merely following the consensus of his era. But I find it very hard to swallow the fact that leaders of the medical establishment can ignore hard evidence of a drug's dangers, blind themselves to new treatment possibilities, and still consider themselves doctors dedicated to the principle, "Do no harm."

For some strange reason the experts, like the lay public, tend to assume automatically that each new drug arriving on the scene is safe. Commenting on this phenomenon, the *New England Journal of Medicine* notes how today's cocaine epidemic is just a rerun of past cycles in the use of stimulant drugs:

> In the 1890s cocaine use surged and was temporarily considered safe; it abated as severe problems of abuse became well known. This pattern was repeated in the 1920s. In the early 1950s and the late 1960s, the same cycle occurred, but the drugs were amphetamine and methamphetamine. [Because there is a time lag between first use of a drug and addiction to it], documentation of abuse during an epidemic first appears several years after premature or naive reports of stimulant safety. The transient illusion of safety has repeatedly enabled serious clinicians and scientists to forget history.

Thus, we now find ourselves in the fifth, and largest, epidemic of stimulant abuse. They might well have added the marijuana epidemic of the 1960s and the tranquilizer plague of the 1970s to their list. Only after we have field-tested the drug on millions of people—and buried more than a few of them—do the experts suddenly smack their foreheads and declare, "Oh, that's right—drugs *are* dangerous, aren't they?"

There's another aspect to the cyclical nature of drug abuse. Almost every *stimulant* epidemic we know of has been followed by an epidemic of *sedative* abuse, as users begin taking "downers" to modulate their intense highs. We're seeing this more and more today, as crack smokers use alcohol, tranquilizers, marijuana, and even smokable or injectable heroin to offset the cocaine rush.

Cocaine isn't safe because Peruvians have used it for centuries or because it was included in the original Coca-Cola. Myths of cocaine's safety fester in the absence of truth. The failure of the experts to recognize and disseminate the facts about drugs has made it possible for fantasy to spread unchecked.

During the sixties, for example, people believed that marijuana was safe and nonaddictive. And given the relatively low THC content of the dope from that era, perhaps only a small percentage of people actually did experience marijuana toxicity or addiction. Now, however, we know that the extremely high THC content of the pot available today makes it a clear health hazard and addictive. But that old myth is pretty hard to dispel, even though we see patients who use it many times a day and who describe themselves as addicted.

Another devastating myth is that "cocaine is safe." This "safe" drug causes high blood pressure, sweating, elevated body temperature, headache, muscle tightening, high blood sugar levels, vitamin depletion, and loss of appetite. It damages your brain, damages your lungs, damages your heart, and causes birth defects. It can lead to sudden death. This is safe? Sometimes I feel like a psychiatric coroner. I do "autopsies" on people who are cocaine casualties. We also study cocaine deaths and see these physical effects and wonder how anyone in his or her right mind would dare promote the notion that cocaine is safe.

"Cocaine is nonaddicting." The experts who touted this idea dismissed the many reports of cocaine dependence as "exaggerations." These geniuses scanned the medical literature, noticed controlled studies on cocaine addiction were scarce, and misinterpreted that fact to mean that cocaine was not addictive. They were even supported in their conclusions with two national commissions on drug abuse, which reported that, yes, amphetamines were dangerous, but not cocaine. I wish they gave a money-back guarantee! Fortunately, the users taught me that cocaine was addicting. Rock stars, business superstars, and 'famous children' flocked to Fair Oaks in great numbers from 1978–1982 for cocaine addictions. To conclude that cocaine wasn't addicting amounted to malpractice. The absence of evidence should never be taken as proof that the opposite case is true. A burglar may leave no fingerprints, but that doesn't prove he's innocent!

One reason the experts reached their faulty conclusions is that they ignored a few inconvenient facts. They ignored the effects of dose, method of administration, and other classic animal studies that clearly showed cocaine being consumed until the animals died. (After struggling with a celebrity who spent $1,000,000 on cocaine, I saw very little difference between monkeys and man.) They even failed to look at emergency room statistics, for example. Had they done so, they might have noticed that between 1976 and 1986 there was a 15-fold increase in the number of emergency room visits due to cocaine and in the number of admissions to public treatment programs for cocaine. Cocaine-related ER visits jumped again by 86 percent in 1987, largely because of the swelling use of crack. Nearly one in four drug-related ER visits involve some combination of drugs and alcohol. By 1989, cocaine was by far the number one cause of drug-related emergency room visits—not just in cities like Washington and New York, but in Atlanta, Baltimore, Chicago, Indianapolis, Detroit, Los Angeles, New Orleans, and many others. We need to be aware of these facts, and make sure everyone knows them, if we intend to educate people and prevent drug use.

The experts also did not have experience with continuous users in the 1970s. They minimized or forgot to consider the long-term effects on babies born to cocaine-addicted mothers. They didn't realize that the number of babies born under the influence of cocaine has risen by a factor of three in most cities. In some parts of the country, as many as one out of every two babies is born under the influence of some illicit drug. We now have to pray for the legions of five-year-old children of crack users, who are hyperactive, have severe learning problems, and have a very questionable future. Such ignorance has meant delays in planning and implementing much-needed programs to reach out to women at high risk of becoming pregnant while using drugs.

As a psychiatrist, I'm appalled at how long it has taken my profession to realize its crucial role in treating drug problems. During my training at Yale in the mid-1970s, the study of drug abuse was not even considered part of the established program in psychiatry. There was no facility for treating addicts on campus. Heaven forbid that junkies should be allowed to wander into the nicer neighborhoods of New Haven! No, they were relegated to shabby treatment houses in some of the bad parts of town. Luckily, I had Herb Kleber. He was tucked away in a small office, begging for someone to teach in return for work. With his help, I had the opportunity to learn about drugs and do my research on drugs after hours, for no credit, in the lousiest parts of the city. I also benefitted from Bob Byck's study on Freud's cocaine papers and David Musto's research into the history of cocaine use. I was detoxifying patients in clinics, jails, in the state hospital for the criminally insane—everywhere, it seemed, but at a clean, well-lighted hospital.

Back then the top brass seemed to think that working with drug addicts was beneath the dignity of psychiatry students. That attitude wasn't limited to Yale; it was common to psychiatry in general. Drugs simply weren't perceived as a psychiatric issue. Addicts were seen as people who didn't pay their bills, who were more likely to whack you over your head than let a shrink get into theirs. Besides, drugs made them talk nonsense. How could you hope to use insight-oriented therapy or talk therapy and make any progress with these spaced-out zombies?

Happily, the situation today is much improved. That's a very significant part of the good news about drugs and alcohol. Attitudes among health care providers about addiction and how to handle it are changing dramatically. The study of substance abuse is now a recognized sub-specialty in psychiatry, similar to cardiology in Internal Medicine. In addition, many of my colleagues have been at the forefront in the battle against drug legalization and in recognizing the need for quality treatments for addiction.

Strangely, though, one of the primary reasons for that change has been an emergence of a powerful therapeutic movement—one led not by professionals, but by addicts themselves.

The name of this movement is Alcoholics Anonymous.

The Insight of AA

Founded in 1935 by Bill Wilson and Dr. Bob Smith—ordinary names for extraordinary men—AA now has two million members around the world. Through its no-nonsense strategy AA has improved, and in many cases actually saved, the lives of millions of people.

The core of AA's philosophy is the justly famous Twelve Step program. These twelve steps promote sobriety through self-help, mutual support, and reinforcement. Underlying all AA activity is a strong spiritual foundation. Although AA is a national, even worldwide, organization, the local self-help networks are run entirely by volunteers who are themselves recovering alcoholics.

To benefit from AA, alcoholics must admit to themselves and to others that they lack the inner power to stay sober. They must recognize that, in a sense, they are permanently disabled—their addiction is incurable, and they are always at risk of readdiction. Thus a sober alcoholic considers himself engaged in a lifelong struggle—always recovering, never recovered—a struggle that has to be faced one day at a time.

As we'll see, the same concepts apply to those who abuse other substances, not just drugs but food as well. For that reason, the Twelve Step concept has been adapted successfully to other programs, including Overeaters Anonymous, Narcotics Anonymous, and Cocaine Anonymous. Because substance abuse is a family issue, groups such as Al-Anon were formed to provide support for those who love and care for the recovering addict.

The AA concept of helplessness derives from perceptive insights into addicts' personalities. Although they often deny it, alcoholics and other substance abusers experience severe psychological problems, including isolation, shame, guilt, and loneliness. Their substance abuse allows them to deny that these unpleasant feelings cause them any trouble in their lives. They are very dependent on outside sources of reinforcement, but as a rule are poor at developing healthy relationships with other people. Given these factors—intense need, painful feelings, reliance on substances to deflect emotional trauma—alcoholics are very often powerless to maintain sobriety under their own steam.

If the problem is seen as a lack of power to control the craving, then the solution comes in drawing power from outside sources. One such source is the love and support shown by fellow alcoholics during AA meetings—as my "12 step" colleagues taught me shortly after my arrival at Fair Oaks in 1978. There is sobriety, as well as safety, in numbers. Unlike much of the outside world, the group accepts the alcoholic despite his or her faults, foibles, and past behavior. Drinkers come to depend on fellow AA members, rather than on alcohol, to fill their emotional needs. Thus the pattern of compulsive substance abuse is replaced by communication, emotional closeness, shared experiences, and the work of helping others regain their equilibrium.

The other main source of power comes from the spirituality embodied in the AA philosophy. For some members, spirituality may mean belief in the orthodox Christian God. For others it may mean something else entirely. Bill Wilson, cofounder of AA, believed that the label given to the source of spirituality was basically irrelevant. What mattered, he wrote, was "being willing to believe in a Power greater than myself. Nothing more was required of me to make my beginning." Although each local AA group tends to develop its own identity—some are more traditionally religious than others—they hold in common a firm belief that the alcoholic must surrender control to a higher power. In AA, surrender is victory.

If you have a friend or a loved one in AA, or if you are a member yourself, you may be a little surprised that a psychiatrist would speak of the organization in such glowing terms. Some people believe the AA approach and that of the medical mainstream are mutually antagonistic. And in many respects that belief is correct. Let me explain.

As a prominent author, addictionologist, and physician, Conway Hunter, points out, doctors are in the business of curing people. AA operates on the principle that addiction *can't* be cured. Thus some doctors may tell their patients, "Stay away from AA. They think you'll never be rid of your problem, that it's hopeless. Stick with me, though, and we'll lick your addiction for good in just a matter of weeks." I've treated hundreds of drug and alcohol addicts, and I know that the AA way of thinking is closer to the mark. Addiction *is* incurable—it's the problem of a lifetime. As we'll learn in the next chapter, many people are actually born with the predisposition to become substance abusers. They carry that trait with them until they die. And if they don't surrender control of their illness to a higher power—God, AA, or even medical treatment—they will die, and sooner rather than later.

Another source of friction is that, almost by definition, the art of medicine involves use of medications. But AA holds that there is no pharmacologic antidote to alcoholism. Relying on drugs to conquer a drug problem is, in the AA view, the wrong approach; better to replace compulsive drug use with commitment to the Twelve Steps and to the other members of the group.

No one individual or group or medical discipline has a lock on the truth. Everybody involved in the fight against drug abuse shares a common desire: to help the person with the problem get better. A recovering person should not automatically reject medical, even pharmacological, help. We will all benefit, patients and caregivers alike, if we share our information and use the best strategies, no matter what their origin, to achieve our goals.

The majority of alcoholics don't need, and will not benefit from, any kind of drug treatment for their drinking problem. The exceptions are those alcoholics who also have some kind of clearly recognizable, organic psychiatric condition, such as manic-depression, which does call for a pharmacological approach. Let me be absolutely clear, though: Use of medications in these circumstances is aimed at correcting the underlying mental disorder, not the alcoholism. By the same token, many people who abuse opiates or cocaine, or who use a combination of drugs and alcohol, *can* benefit from the use of medications and from certain psychiatric therapies.

But when caregivers, lay as well as professional, draw from the best of both worlds, the psychiatric and the Twelve Step, they give the substance abuser the best chance of improving. I'll go even further: Any medical drug treatment program in 1991 that fails to include a Twelve Step strategy is not a serious program and simply will not work. Period.

The success of AA has forced doctors to reassess their notions of what substance abuse really is. Another force for change has been the growing emergence of a revolutionary form of psychiatry that focuses on the biological causes of mental disorders. I'll devote the rest of this chapter to this innovative medical discipline known as biopsychiatry.

Biopsychiatry

As I mentioned in an earlier chapter, part of my training at Yale involved the then-new science of neurobiology, the study of interactions between the brain and the body. In addition to my mentors, I was supervised by a host of dedicated teachers and researchers who were true pioneers in this field, from George Heninger ("Psychiatric diagnosis is a '57 VW") to John Flynn ("Stimulate this electrode and watch") to James Maas ("Biochemical subgroups of depression exist") to Don Sweeney ("Panic attacks are physical. No one could wish this kind of stuff upon themselves") to Bob Davies ("You do not have to have a motor convulsion to have a seizure or an electrical malfunction in the brain causing thinking problems") to Dave Pickar ("You couldn't have picked a better time to enter psychiatry") to Boris Astrachan ("This isn't backbiting, this is academic psychiatry . . . Do the research and empower the public with accurate information") to Andrew Slaby ("Examine the patient first, then get a urine, then ask everyone involved what drugs he has been taking"). In my enthusiasm for the subject, I felt a compelling urge to apply neurobiologic discoveries to the practice of psychiatry. Whenever I had doubts or needed a rescue from a research dead end, Herb Kleber, Gene Redmond or Bob Byck chipped in with a new idea to consider.

At that time, a decade and a half or so ago, psychiatry had fallen into a state of near-total disarray. Why? Basically because those who practiced psychiatry had forgotten, literally, where their heads were at. They ignored the neurobiological fact that their heads—and those of their patients, for that matter—were attached to bodies. To separate the two, and assume that mental disorders had little or no connection to what was happening elsewhere in the body, caused psychiatry to lose a lot of ground.

As Bob Byck pointed out psychiatrists as a group had forgotten their roots in the practice of medicine. They set aside all their years of training in anatomy, biochemistry, and physiology —the same training all doctors of medicine receive—and focused instead on the psychodynamic or "all-in-the-head" aspects of mental illness. For most of the century, psychiatrists, following the pattern set by their teachers, chose to ignore the role that brain diseases and disruptions in other organ systems play in causing emotional symptoms.

The situation grew worse in the 1960s. Karl Menninger, founder of the Menninger Clinic in Topeka, Kansas, published an influential book, *The Vital Balance,* in which he lumped all mental afflictions together as one disorder. That being so, he argued, all mental illness will respond to one technique: psychotherapy, the "talking cure" that relies on deep introspection to reveal the unconscious motivations behind the patient's behavior. (Brandon, whom we met earlier, ran into this therapeutic brick wall with his psychiatrist.) At around the same time another psychiatrist, Thomas Szasz, published *The Myth of Mental Illness,* the title of which reveals his notion that there wasn't even one form of mental affliction. Like the man without a country, psychiatrists become doctors without a disease.

As psychiatry lost ground, other types of professionals were happy to fill the void. Psychologists, social workers, exercise therapists, artists, and other people, usually with no formal medical training, not allowed to dispense medicines, tried, often vainly, to help patients who in most cases were suffering from physical illnesses.

The 1970s saw a change. Many important new medications became available for the treatment of mental diseases. For example, a class of drugs known as tricyclic antidepressants (such as Elavil and Tofranil) helped end the suffering for some people who experienced debilitating periods of low mood. Having a new tool to work with also lifted the spirits of psychiatrists who, frustrated by the poor results of talk therapy, felt thwarted in their efforts to help severely depressed or anxious patients (and who were rapidly losing business to the less expensive nonmedical therapists).

Enthusiastic psychiatrists, however, tended to overprescribe these medications. The so-called "minor" tranquilizers, prescribed for patients who displayed the slightest hint of anxiety, turned out to be addicting. Other antidepressant medications were available, but we psychiatrists seemed to only prescribe Elavil for everyone who wasn't on Valium. Antipsychotic drugs produced permanent side effects, such as involuntary movements of the face and tongue. Public outcry was such that some doctors erred in the other direction, failing to prescribe these medications even when they were likely to do some good. It was a classic double bind: Psychiatrists couldn't win for losing.

It takes a long time to get a clear picture of whether certain medical treatments work. Now, after years of experience with the new psychiatric medications, the results are in: They do and don't. Miracle drugs produce no miracles. Antidepressants have about the same rate of success as cognitive therapy (therapy aimed at changing disturbed patterns of thinking). Together the two approaches are better than either alone. Many who seem cured relapse within a year or six months. In fact, five or six out of ten people with depression will get better on their own, without ever consulting a doctor.

My course of training had helped me to recognize what the problem with modern psychiatry was. It wasn't that the treatments had failed. The practitioners had failed to remember their backgrounds and apply treatment in a rigorous, scientific way. They relied too much on trial and error and neglected the science.

Like all drugs, antidepressants work by changing body chemistry and function. Yes, an antidepressant can be effective —if you can identify the patient whose depression springs from a biological malfunction, not from some disturbing situation such as a death in the family. If you've correctly identified such patients, but aren't seeing the response you predicted, the problem may be in the dosage. We've treated hundreds of so-called "untreatable" patients and found that just by tinkering with their doses we can send them home happy and healthy. Both therapy and medicine together are better than either alone. To spot the patients who will respond to various treatments, and to monitor the results of therapy, you must make full use of standardized interviews and diagnostic methods like blood levels tests—those vital tools that "real" doctors use every day, but that psychiatrists seem to neglect.

Part of the good news, then, is that more and more treatment professionals are returning to their origins and applying the rigorous standards of science and medicine to the practice of psychiatry.

The results in just a short time have been nothing short of phenomenal. Within a few years, biopsychiatry has uncovered evidence that many patients with depression do indeed have another illness or a brain disease or some other specific and identifiable malfunction—a thyroid problem, for example—that mimics psychiatric mood disorders. We are keenly aware of the relationship between genetics and psychiatric illness, and are working to figure out which biological, psychosocial, or environmental factors might cause the illness to develop. We see how the body's endocrine system, responsible for releasing a cascade of powerful hormones, can disrupt mental equilibrium, and how emotional turmoil can disrupt the immune system's ability to fight off infections or other disease.

Such findings aren't mere speculation. We can demonstrate them under the microscope, in test tubes, and on the flickering screens of powerful devices that allow us to peer inside the living body and brain.

Nor are the new psychiatrists just an isolated handful of mavericks, trying to foment rebellion from our outposts in a few far-flung hospitals and clinics. I used to be avant-garde, now I'm told that I've become almost boringly mainstream.

Our greatest accomplishment has been to reestablish psychiatry as a legitimate branch of medicine. Recently in its manual of therapeutics and updates the American Psychiatric Association stressed the value of using all of the various tools available today for psychiatric diagnosis and treatment. Educators in medical schools now train future psychiatrists to obtain careful patient histories, conduct complete physical exams, and order all the necessary lab workups—just like "real" doctors! Although there is still much room for improvement in drug and alcohol terminology, the latest edition of the psychiatrist's "bible," the *Diagnostic and Statistical Manual,* reflects some of the new understanding on substance abuse in its descriptions of addiction and its symptoms. Clinical procedures and data collection and analysis have been improved. In short, the biopsychiatric explosion has led to a much greater awareness of the interplay among the biological, neurological, psychological, and social aspects of psychiatry.

I use the term "biopsychiatry" to describe this important movement. In reality, *all* psychiatry should be—and one day will be—biopsychiatry.

Unfortunately, while traditional psychiatry has dramatically improved its diagnosis and treatment of substance abuse, there is still room for improvement. Preparations for the next installment of the *Diagnostic and Statistical Manual,* called DSM-IV, indicate a continuation of the failure to consider urine or blood tests in diagnosing substance abuse. It is puzzling that the DSM-IV will most likely ignore the diagnostic tools used by the police (Breathalyzers), coroners (blood tests), and sports team physicians (urine tests.) Traditional reluctance to embrace these proven diagnostic tools baffles me.

Biopsychiatry and Drug Abuse

Biopsychiatrists, having made great strides in the treatment of depression and anxiety, are now applying their skills to the problem of drug and alcohol addiction. Let me share with you some of what we've learned.

One vital lesson, gleaned from the experience of Alcoholics Anonymous, is that chemical dependency is not the result of a person's moral failure. Nor is it a sin, a crime, a form of divine punishment, a sign of weakness, or anyone's fault. *It is a disease.* Substance abuse is a physical problem with emotional consequences, and not the other way around. We don't point a finger at a person with arthritis and say "You are crippled because you are morally unfit." We don't go around blaming someone for having diabetes. Neither should we look at people who need help overcoming an addiction and accuse them of "lacking willpower" or being "unfit for society."

If dependency is a disease, then how is it transmitted? There are several pathways.

In many cases people inherit the tendency to become substance abusers. Research on families of alcoholics confirms that having a family history of alcohol abuse increases the risk of developing alcoholism by as much as 50 percent. Similar patterns are seen among families in which a member abuses substances other than alcohol, such as cocaine or narcotics. It even appears that, for perhaps one out of every ten people, addiction is biologically inevitable. I'll describe in more detail the studies that led to these conclusions in the next section of this book.

Another biological factor has to do with the body's ability to regulate itself. The body has a number of "thermostats" to keep things working smoothly. These thermostats are programmed to protect the body against excessive weight loss or gain, temperature change and so on. If, for example, your weight drops below a certain level, the weight regulator in your brain will kick in, shutting down some systems and accelerating others in an effort to get you to eat more.

This fascinating concept, known as the "set point" theory, applies to the study of substance abuse as well. People have different set points that determine their vulnerability to drugs or alcohol. A shot of whiskey might have no impact whatsoever on Jill, whereas Jack might drink the same amount, fall down, and break his crown. Everybody's physiology is different. Some people can metabolize (break down) toxic substances better or more efficiently than others. Our set points are part of our genetic inheritance. We can set the thermostats in our homes to higher or lower temperatures; we can't, however, change our set points.

If you have a low set point for cocaine metabolism, then even a small dose might overwhelm your body's defenses, invade delicate tissues, and damage brain cells. As we'll discuss in Chapter Seven, such damage can affect the neurotransmitter systems and cause your body to desire drugs in the same way it desires food and sex. A few snorts can set people with a low set point threshold for drug tolerance on the path to addiction.

There's more to the problem than genetics, however. You might have inherited a gene for obesity, but if you live on a desert island where there is very little food, you probably won't ever get fat. Likewise, if you are born predisposed to substance abuse, you won't suffer from the disease if you never have access to drugs or alcohol.

Another way that addiction is "transmitted," then, is through social contact. The sheer availability of alcohol in our society—it's legal, heavily promoted, and an integral part of many of our customs and rituals—puts liquor into the hands of people who may not be able to handle it. The glamorization of drugs in our culture makes drug use seem like the thing to do, especially to vulnerable adolescents and children who lack the maturity of judgment to see the risks involved. Too often our society sends a message that problems can be cured instantly. Pop a pill, and boom—all is well.

Biopsychiatry has helped untangle the knotty relationships between substance abuse and other psychiatric illnesses. The debate revolves around cause versus effect. For example, does a mood disorder *cause* someone to use drugs as a form of self-medication? Or is the mood disorder an *effect* of drug use? The answer, from a biopsychiatric standpoint, is a little bit of both. I've seen all types: patients who had depression and used drugs as a means of coping with their low mood; patients whose drug use *led* to disturbances in mood; and patients who had *both* a mood disorder and a concurrent problem with substance abuse.

Study after study confirms that many people with psychiatric disorders are also substance abusers. A national study of over 20,000 Americans found that 13.5 percent developed an alcohol problem or addiction during their lifetime and 6.1 percent another drug dependence or addiction. Of those individuals with an alcohol problem, 37 percent also had another psychiatric condition; among those with another drug problem, 53 percent also suffered a psychiatric disorder. Other researchers have found that as many as 87 percent of drug addicts experience a psychiatric disorder—not counting their addiction—at some time in their lives. Roughly half of these will have major depression; one in four will have antisocial personalities; and one in ten suffers from some kind of phobia. About 15 percent of adolescent substance abusers turn out to have depression; up to 20 percent have (or had at one time) an attention deficit/hyperactivity syndrome.

Interestingly, there seems to be a connection between a person's mental disorder and his drug of choice. For example, those who use stimulants, such as cocaine and amphetamines, are more likely to experience moods that swing from very high to very low (known in psychiatry as a bipolar disorder, because moods shift between two extremes, or "poles.") In fact, in the

1970s, the similarity between the manic swings of a bipolar disorder and the high and subsequent crash of a cocaine abuser led Bob Byck and I to postulate that the manic high of a bipolar patient might be caused by a cocainelike substance. Opiate abusers, on the other hand, show higher rates of major depression. Alcoholics are more prone to panic, anxiety, and phobia.

As I indicated, the presence of a psychiatric disturbance can lead a person to drug or alcohol dependence. Evaluating a case in the Yale emergency room with Drew Slaby in 1976 made this point very clear. Bipolar patients often drank alcohol to try to control their mania. Only after their drunkenness wore off would they "look manic" and respond to treatment with lithium. In such cases, the addiction is really secondary to the underlying illness. Biopsychiatrists are alert to this fact, and also know that many seemingly mental disorders have physical causes. Thus they are more likely to perceive a person's chemical dependency as a sign of a deeper problem.

A case in point is Ariel, who came to Fair Oaks following years of unsuccessful attempts at treating her depression. Antidepressants hadn't worked; analysis hadn't worked. "All the other psychiatrists just gave up," she told me. For the past year or so Ariel had tried to treat herself and lift her moods, first through alcohol, then cocaine, and now she uses both a few times a week.

"Did anything show up on your physical exam?" I asked.

"I don't know," she replied. "I haven't had one for years."

I could barely suppress my surprise. "You mean *none* of your psychiatrists did a physical? Did any schedule you to see an internist or other specialist?" She shook her head. "But I did have a physical a while back. They told me I should lose some weight."

I immediately took her pulse and blood pressure, felt her hair and neck, and ordered a series of tests, the results of which confirmed my suspicion: Ariel suffered from hypothyroidism. Her thyroid, a gland in the neck, was enlarged. The thyroid secretes hormones that control body metabolism. One result of having too low a supply of thyroid hormone is a mood disturbance that looks for all the world like major depression but that is really just a reversible chemical imbalance. All these years Ariel had been treated for depression. Her attempts at self-medication had then led to a substance abuse problem. It turns out all that she needed was therapy with a supplemental thyroid hormone.

No amount of antidepressant medication, no outpatient program or four-week stay at a cocaine detox clinic would have done anything to correct the biological malfunction that lay at the root of Ariel's problem. By taking a biopsychiatric approach, I saw beyond the outward signs and symptoms and uncovered the real, physical cause of her illness. Once that was accomplished, I was able to choose a form of treatment—simple, effective, inexpensive, and quick—that addressed her needs.

Biopsychiatry to the rescue!

CHAPTER FOUR

Addiction Is . . .

Want to start an argument? Just ask a roomful of psychiatrists to define addiction.

"Addiction is clearly a conditioned response," says the Behavioral Psychiatrist.

"Addiction results from a learned behavior," says the Cognitive Psychiatrist.

"Addiction results from a dysfunctional family," says the Family Therapy Psychiatrist.

"Addiction is biological," says the Research Psychiatrist.

"You are all right," says the Biopsychiatrist, "and you are all wrong. And we have much more to learn."

Addiction is so difficult a concept that even the World Health Organization (WHO) has struggled (vainly, I might add) to define it. The WHO has even suggested that the phrase "drug abuse" not be used since "abuse" has negative connotations (of course it has negative connotations—it *should* have negative connotations. After all, we are discussing some very powerful and dangerous drugs, not afternoon tea with crumpets).

At the risk of offending the WHO and countless other "experts," let me offer my definition, a definition that is crucial to *The Good News About Drugs and Alcohol:*

Addiction is a disease characterized by repetitive and destructive use of one or more mood-altering substances, and stems from a biological vulnerability exposed or induced by environmental forces.

This statement is bound to stir up a little controversy among professionals and nonprofessionals alike. So, allow me to explain this definition in greater detail.

The Most Important Medical Discovery of the Twentieth Century

Name the most important medical discovery of the twentieth century? Penicillin? The Polio Vaccine? X rays?

In my personal and professional opinion one of the most important discoveries is the statement: *Addiction is a disease.* This statement has helped millions of people to stop blaming themselves for their illness, allowing them to take that first step to recovery. To many people today this statement is obvious, something they've heard a million times on countless talk shows and movies-of-the-week. But 50 years ago, even 20 years ago, I would have been laughed out of medical school for even suggesting such a preposterous notion.

Until recently, addicts were seen as people who were morally unfit and lacking in willpower. Their cravings were only figments of their imaginations, a sign of mental weakness. If they could just "pull themselves together," they could lick their problem. Addicts were "losers." They had no self-control, couldn't face reality, and were afraid of their emotions or of responsibility. Didn't the frequent failure of treatment—whether psychoanalysis or some other form—just prove how much of a loser the addict really was?

As we saw in the previous chapter, the insights provided by AA and others who wrestled with addiction have changed our perceptions completely. Unfortunately, medicine's failure to initially understand addiction has made many recovering people suspicious of the medical profession. On numerous occasions recovering addicts have asked me about my own drug use. When I tell them that I have never used cocaine or suffered from alcoholism, they usually respond with something like, "How can you be a cocaine expert?" or, "Well, only a recovering addict can really help another addict." This attitude, while understandable 30 years ago, ignores the many valuable achievements medicine and psychiatry have made within the last 20 years. A person in recovery who shuns the contributions of the medical profession is just as bad as the doctor who ignores the valuable insights provided by recovering people.

For the first time in human history both professionals and non-professionals understand a crucial fact: Addiction is a disease.

But this statement isn't enough; good medicine and good science demand that the statement "addiction is a disease" be proven. First, every disease must have a physical basis, even if the exact nature of its physical origin is unknown. There are several factors that support the biological basis of addiction:

1. *Inheritability.* Any disorder that can be passed from one generation to the next clearly has a biological basis. To establish the genetic basis of addiction, researchers conducted studies of twins involving both identical and fraternal twins. Unlike fraternal twins, identical twins share the same genetic makeup and are essentially genetic clones of each other. A major study of identical twins found that if one twin was an alcoholic, there was a 74 percent chance that the other twin would also be an alcoholic. However, among fraternal twins there was only a 32 percent chance of each twin being an alcoholic. Other twin studies supported these findings.

Critics challenged these studies, claiming that, when compared to fraternal twins, identical twins are socially closer and therefore more likely to influence each other. Subsequent studies did establish that identical twins are socially closer, but that this closeness still could not fully explain the similarities between the alcoholic twins.

An even more compelling argument in favor of the inheritability of addiction came from adoption studies. Several adoption studies have shown that children born to alcoholic parents but adopted during infancy and raised by nonalcoholic, adoptive parents were more likely to become alcoholics than children born to nonalcoholic parents. Adoption studies are important because they clearly show the importance of genetics regardless of the environmental factors.

No matter how compelling, these twin and adoption studies by themselves would not be sufficient to establish the physical basis of addiction. Fortunately, I have several more arguments to offer.

2. *Animal Studies.* Some lay people, especially *uneducated* lay people, ridicule animal studies claiming (in so many words) that animals are no substitutes for human beings. In reality, studies of rats and mice have been essential in improving our understanding of addiction. For example, researchers have been able to selectively breed both mice and rats, creating strains of rodents that differ in their reaction—and in their attraction—to alcohol, cocaine, and opiates.

In the laboratory, rodent strains have been bred according to their *preference* for alcohol (called P rats) or their dislike for alcohol (called *nonpreference* or NP rats.) The P rats appear to be alcoholics: They voluntarily consume and work to get enough alcohol to make themselves drunk even when there is sufficient food and water available. Conversely, the NP rats could care less about alcohol.

Studies of the P and NP rats reveal significant physical differences between the two groups. In one study, scientists gave low amounts of alcohol to both groups and then measured brain activity with electroencephalograms (EEGs). The EEGs revealed that the NP rats were mildly sedated by the alcohol (a normal reaction since alcohol is a depressant) but that the P rats were stimulated by the alcohol! This stimulation could possibly explain the attractiveness of alcohol to P rats.

Neurochemical differences between the two rodent groups also occur. These differences even appear in P and NP rats that have never consumed alcohol (further strengthening the genetic argument). Studies of these neurochemical differences have focused on substances called neurotransmitters (neurotransmitters are the chemical messengers between cells). The P rats have reduced levels of two essential neurotransmitters called serotonin and dopamine. Both serotonin and dopamine are essential in humans for regulating moods, with reduced serotonin levels being associated with depression, irritability, and aggression. In fact, a very popular antidepressant medication called Prozac (generic name fluoxetine) works by enhancing the availability of serotonin. Interestingly, when Prozac is given to the alcohol-preferring rats it reduces their alcohol consumption—a finding that may be shown to have tremendous significance for humans.

Genetic studies of P and NP strains have even suggested that a specific genetic marker may be responsible for the alcoholic rodents. According to one theory, variations in a specific gene that produces a protein found in the brain, liver, and kidney of mice may be responsible for the P mice affinity for alcohol. A variation of this gene occurs in the alcohol-preferring mice, but not in the non-preferring group.

Mice are nice, but what about genetic markers in humans? Genetic markers in humans are notoriously difficult to identify. Difficult, but not impossible. Seemingly every day major breakthroughs add to our understanding of our genetic material. Recently, for example, a variation of a specific gene by-product—in this case, the human brain protein with the catchy name of PC-1 Duarte—has been identified with increased frequency in populations of alcoholics. A recent report—confirmed by other studies—suggests that the dopamine D2 receptor gene occurs significantly more frequently in alcoholics than in nonalcoholics.

Obviously much work remains to establish a definitive marker for addiction. In a later chapter I will examine future directions in genetic research in greater detail, as well as discuss the possible importance of identifying individuals at risk for addiction. However, for now I will continue my discussion of the biological basis of addiction by focusing on the addict's physical response to alcohol and drugs.

3. *The Addict's Body Is Different.* How does a doctor know if a patient is suffering from diabetes? The patient complains of excessive thirst, frequent urination, and other problems the doctor associates with diabetes—a clinical hunch in need of confirmation. The most common way of confirming a diabetes diagnosis involves a glucose tolerance test (GTT). In the GTT, a small amount of glucose is administered while the patient's response to the sugar is monitored. Diabetics respond differently than nondiabetics, hence the GTT can confirm a diagnosis of diabetes.

While we lack the definitiveness of the GTT, researchers have discovered that the physical responses of addicts differ from nonaddicts. One study using EEG measurement of brain activity found that, compared to the general public, sons of alcoholics are more sensitive to moderate doses of alcohol. Another study of male drug abusers found that slower EEG and brainstem response was associated with antisocial and aggressive behavior—two characteristics that have been associated with substance abuse. Other studies have found that alcoholics, even abstinent alcoholics, responded more slowly to visual or auditory clues when compared to nonalcoholics.

These findings suggest that the brains of alcoholics process information differently. This conclusion is supported by various studies conducted at alcohol and drug treatment facilities, which report that between 45 and 70 percent of their patients have specific deficits in problem solving, abstract thinking, and memory. It's not certain whether these problems reflect a genetic vulnerability, or the effects of years of addiction, or a combination of the two.

Twin studies, adoptive studies, animal studies, genetic markers, and EEGs have all underscored the biological nature of addiction. Remember the good old days of the sixties when college students used to argue about "physical versus psychological addiction"? Well, in this new age of biopsychiatry, we've reattached the head and the body, and in so doing have begun to make real progress in fighting the disease.

Seeing addiction as a disease helps us realize that it is a chronic and relapsing illness. Alcoholics Anonymous taught the world that the substance abuser is always at risk of reverting to old habits. Recovery is a lifelong process, with the ever-present possibility of relapse. A crack addict who has been drug-free for 18 months in an intensive residential program might still go back to the pipe within days of release. Recognizing this truth lets us focus treatment on the real needs of addicts, rather than on the fantasy of purging the addict's demons forever.

Another advantage of the disease model of addiction is that it underscores the real cause of the problem: not the specific chemical of abuse, but the individual's susceptibility and reactions to that chemical.

For example, some people are allergic to pollen. You might try to prevent allergies by wiping out every plant on the planet. But that's not very practical. You have a much better chance of prevention if you identify the people who are vulnerable to pollen. You can then teach these people how to avoid it, or at least how to minimize the damage should they come in contact with it.

The same can be said of addiction. By recognizing how people fall into drug abuse, we can show them how to keep from using drugs in the first place. This method—education for prevention—has a lot better chance of working than trying to eliminate chemicals.

Addiction is a progressive disease. And unless the addict gets help, it's also a fatal one.

The Stages of Addiction

The disease model—conceiving of addiction as a biological illness—allows us to trace the course of the illness, just as we trace the course of pneumonia or a common cold. It's clear that addicts pass through certain stages on their way to total chemical dependency. If we can recognize those stages, we can intervene sooner, provide appropriate treatment, and prevent a problem from becoming a tragedy.

The first stage of addiction is known as the "experimental" stage. This involves occasional, spontaneous use of beer or marijuana, usually at weekend parties among peers. Most people go through this phase as adolescents.

Passage into the next stage occurs when the person starts using the drug alone, often before going to school or work. This is when *tolerance* develops; someone who at first got plastered on two beers or wiped out on half a joint now needs more of the drug just to feel the same effect.

Biologically, there are two reasons why tolerance occurs. First, on one level the body's ability to metabolize a drug (the process of breaking down and eliminating a substance) improves with repeated exposure to a drug. The body simply becomes more efficient at removing the drug; hence the drug's effects are reduced. Second, with prolonged exposure to a drug, individual cells become less sensitive to concentrations of the drug in the blood. For these reasons, the user needs more and more of the drug to achieve the effects that he has become accustomed to.

At the third stage, drug use takes over more of the person's time and energy. Solitary use becomes more frequent. The need for money to support the habit means that many users turn to dealing. Others steal from parents, employers, even friends. Many people who reach this point notice that drugs are beginning to interfere with their lives—they may get into trouble at school or with the law.

It isn't a very big leap to the final stage: dependency. At this point the person uses drugs daily, finding it very hard to skip a day. The physical side effects of the drug cause problems. Alcohol and drugs like cocaine squelch the desire to eat; many users become malnourished and suffer from medical complications and nutritional deficiencies. Poor nutrition weakens the whole system, making it susceptible to diseases. Addicts who use needles to inject their drugs risk contracting life-threatening infections ranging from hepatitis to AIDS.

For people in this final stage, drugs become the whole focus of their lives. They form relationships only with other users or with dealers. Their only pleasurable activities revolve around drug use. In the early stages, people using drugs report that they get a short-lived, pleasurable buzz. Further along, however, they use them more to ward off the unpleasant feelings of "rebound" or withdrawal. Those who are cocaine dependent, for example, admit they often snort coke not to feel good but to keep themselves from feeling bad.

Another trait of this stage, as I mentioned, is denial. I can't tell you how many times I've looked into addicts' eyes and listened as they said, "Drugs are no problem for me. I'm in control."

To summarize these stages: Use leads to tolerance; tolerance to abuse; abuse to chemical dependence and addiction.

The Pathways of Addiction

The process by which someone becomes addicted is a complex one. In a sense, the process begins if, at the moment of conception, the person-to-be inherits a family tendency toward substance abuse. Other physiological factors—the chemical environment in the uterus, or inherited supplies of certain brain chemicals, for example—may also come into play. So does a person's medical history—diseases, surgery, use of medications. Some of the psychological factors contributing to substance abuse include low self-esteem, guilt, and loneliness. The emotional environment in the home plays a part too. Once drug use begins, the very nature of the drug itself contributes to the severity of the problem.

Evidence from an exciting avenue of research suggests that the addictive drive, and the body's responses to chemicals, are controlled by a part of the brain called the limbic system. We still have much to learn about this system. We know, however, that it is, in evolutionary terms, a very old part of the brain. In fact, the limbic system in humans is not much different from that found in primitive mammals.

Part of the limbic system—actually a kind of "brain within the brain"—contains nerve cells that help regulate moods. Another part arouses or modulates feelings ranging from joy to misery, and from love to hate. Some limbic structures are involved with memory processing, while others help us perceive a sense of reward. (Reward, in this context, means the body's way of telling us that we've done something right. For example, we have to eat to live; our body rewards us by making eating a pleasurable experience, thus reinforcing our eating behavior and helping assure our survival, both as individuals and as a species.)

Drugs work by changing the ways the brain responds to stimuli. Because it is involved in so many basic functions, the limbic system appears to be particularly vulnerable to drugs. Some drugs, for example, trigger the "reward" response. The body is tricked into thinking, "Hey, cocaine makes me feel great! That drug must be necessary for my survival. Give me more!" In this way, use of a drug stimulates even more use. To make things worse, the limbic system then files this pleasurable response into its nearby memory banks. At some level, then, the brain is prone to think: "Gee, remember how nice that drug made me feel? Maybe I'd better signal this body to get ahold of some more." Basic research is providing some clues that different drugs of abuse may have persisted through the years because they share a common effect on brain-reward chemicals. Even though they are different chemicals acting on different brain receptors, cocaine and heroin may actually be very much alike.

With repeated use, drug and alcohol use becomes what scientists call "entrained" behavior, as easily and spontaneously triggered as our desire to eat, drink, or have sex. The trouble is that these same drugs affect another part of the brain—the frontal lobe—which leads to impaired judgment and lack of insight. So here we have a person with a brain, one part of which has been conditioned to seek reward through the use of dangerous drugs, and another part of which has lost the ability to think clearly and exercise common sense. That, my friends, is a formula for disease.

The changes in the brain that I've just described can occur in anyone, given enough of a drug over a long period of time. But I estimate that, on the average, one person out of ten is born already predisposed to become dependent on drugs or alcohol. That figure changes depending on such factors as family history and the drug involved.

Drugs can addict anyone, but some may be more vulnerable. Recent studies of marijuana indicate that, in a genetically predisposed person, addiction to THC can begin almost immediately. Addicts and nonaddicts alike may start using marijuana for the same reasons: to elevate their moods, as part of social rituals, or at parties. Someone who is not predisposed to addiction may be able to stop using the drug. Because of their genetic vulnerability, however, addicts are unable to stop, regardless of the consequences. As part of the plan to educate young people, we need to emphasize one point very strongly: A person's predisposition to become addicted can't be detected until drug use has begun. *And by then it's too late.*

Because the body and the brain are such complex structures, it would be wrong to say that there is only one clear-cut pathway to addiction. Even people with no predisposition or family history of addiction can become addicts. A substance abuse disorder, like any psychiatric disorder, many result from a disturbance in any of several systems.

Let me explain. If you are General Motors, your ability to roll a new car off the assembly line depends on having a lot of things happen in just the right sequence. But if your shipment of steel is delayed, the parts aren't delivered, your assembly equipment breaks down, or your work force goes on strike, the result is the same: no new cars. By the same token, one person may experience a breakdown in a neurotransmitter system, while another has a metabolic disorder and another suffers from extreme physical and emotional responses to stress. In each of these cases, however, the result may be the same: chemical dependency.

Some people reading this book may think, "Swell. Drug abuse is hard-wired into our bodies. Then how can we hope to fight addiction if we're born with a tendency toward substance abuse? Isn't that like trying to wipe out some physical trait, like brown hair?"

Not at all. Part of the good news I want to share is that *biology is not destiny.* For one thing, just because you inherited a certain gene does not necessarily mean you will express the trait that gene is coded for. People programmed to develop diabetes, for example, can often keep the disease at bay through careful diet and exercise. The same is true for inherited psychiatric illnesses; one study found that only about 60 percent of the people with the genetic tendency toward manic depression actually developed the illness.

This suggests that if people control their behavior and their environment they may be able to prevent the genetic tendency to abuse substances from taking control of their lives. Even if the problem does emerge, they may be able to control its severity. In both instances, education, prevention, and treatment are key steps to take along the path away from addiction.

There is some evidence that, in certain cases, the addict's choice of drugs may be a matter of circumstance. If some cocaine users can't get coke, they'll use alcohol. Take that away, and in a little while they'll discover Valium or Xanax. Keep them away from those drugs and they'll find speed. The list, I'm sorry to say, is endless and need not be limited to drugs. Research from the Eating Disorders Center at Fair Oaks Hospital has shown that in some cases, bulimia and anorexia may be a form of addiction to food and may affect the same parts of the brain that drugs do. For that matter, any kind of behavior that overstimulates the brain's reward centers—chain smoking, gambling, jogging, even video-game playing—can result in addictive behavior: compulsion, loss of control, and disregard for harmful consequences.

Thus a person who tends to get hooked on one drug must

also abstain from all other drugs with the potential for abuse. At Fair Oaks we teach our patients that a recovering coke addict can't become a social drinker. (Many of our "celebrity" patients from the 1970s and early 1980s rejected this message. Fortunately, many had learned enough to seek out help from AA or an alcohol rehab center after they switched from cocaine to alcohol and/or marijuana.) The recovering heroin addict can't smoke an occasional joint. The message we must get across is simple: Addiction is addiction is addiction.

In this chapter I've focused heavily on the biological basis of addiction, as well as the patterns the disease follows as it develops. But as anyone who has struggled with the flu can tell you, it is the symptoms of the disorder that make our lives miserable. No definition of addiction can be complete without a thorough understanding of these symptoms.

What Are the Symptoms of Addiction?

Listen to Whittaker, a 32-year-old airline mechanic: "I remember one Sunday night driving back from my in-laws. I got my wife and two kids in the car. Suddenly I'm driving down this side street, way out of the way. I tell my wife I gotta pick up a newspaper. I leave them sitting in the car and run into this building, where they got a crack house on the second floor. My wife and kids are in the car double-parked and I'm upstairs getting high. My God, I loved that pipe more than anything, more than my family. Some life, huh?"

Here's Amber, a 25-year-old ambulance dispatcher: "I'd wake up in the morning feeling like dog breath. I would tell myself, 'That's it, no more, you're killing yourself. You can't do that much cocaine every night and expect to live like a human being.' But then midway through the day I'd start to feel this craving. I'd think, 'One line, that's all. Then I'll stop.' I'd rummage around in my purse—I somehow never bothered to take the stuff out and just leave it home. I'd pop into the john, toot up, and feel fine for a while. Then I started making more and more trips to the bathroom, and each time I'd do a line, or maybe two or three. When my shift was over I wouldn't even eat dinner. I just wanted coke. I told myself I knew what I was doing, that I could stop anytime, that I was in control."

Kipp, 18 years old: "My parents said if they ever found out I used drugs they'd kick me out of the house. I was becoming careless. I'd been stealing their booze since I was 13 and I figured I could get away with anything. My mom was putting away laundry and she found my stash. Dad threw all my stuff into boxes on the front porch and changed the locks. 'We warned you,' he said. I went to live with my brother for a while. I had to make some money—had to pay rent, and I needed to get high to cope with all the tension. I started dealing a little. Once a cop saw me. He said he wouldn't arrest me this time because he knew my dad and it was my first offense. But if he caught me again, he'd come down on me, and hard. The next day I was back at it. Got busted. You'd think I'd have learned."

Whittaker, Amber, Kipp—their stories, like those of hundreds of other patients I've met over the years, are just part of the big addiction picture.

An addictive disease has five main symptoms:

- compulsion
- loss of control
- preoccupation with the drug
- continued use despite adverse consequences
- denial

A *compulsion* is a persistent and overwhelming need to do something, even if that "something" works against your own best interests. We saw an example of compulsion in Whittaker's story. As he told me, "I loved that pipe more than anything."

Loss of control is a somewhat misleading phrase. A drug user never really has much control to lose. As Amber discovered, she couldn't control her habit. Oh, she might hold out for a few hours. Pretty soon, though, her daily use rose until she could think of nothing but how to get more of the drug. As she recalled, "You don't control coke. Coke controls you. Trying to control that urge was like making a dam out of sugar cubes. Your resistance dissolves and crumbles in no time at all."

One clue that drug use is out of control is if the amount and frequency of the dose keeps climbing. Two joints a week become four, then ten, then two joints a day. The use of crack "just to get a rush at a weekend party" becomes a $200-a-day nightmare. That "quick drink after work" triggers a binge. When I hear someone say they need their drug "just to function normally," I know the problem has already spiralled out of control.

Not long ago I spoke with a patient named Salem who told me that he couldn't possibly be an alcoholic.

"Why is that?" I asked.

"Because I haven't had a drink in two years," he replied proudly.

"Do you ever wish you could have a drink?"

"God, yes. Every time I pass a bar I think about it. But I just grit my teeth and move on."

I told Salem that what he was describing was a classic case of alcoholism. You see, he was the victim of a common misunderstanding: Addiction does not mean the uncontrolled use of drugs or alcohol. It means that *the need for control is always there, every day, 24 hours a day.* Salem thought he wasn't an alcoholic because he had not succumbed to the temptation to drink. On the contrary, he was an alcoholic precisely because the temptation to lose control was always present.

Another aspect of addiction is the *preoccupation* users have with their substance of choice. If you've ever spoken to an addict for any length of time, you become amazed at—and profoundly bored by—how focused they are on their drug. They prattle endlessly about the quality of the stuff, or what they have to do to get it, or how they feel and think while high. They're like a TV set that only picks up one channel, and that one channel only carries one program, endlessly repeated. All of their mental and physical energy is directed toward one end: finding and using the drug.

Kipp's story illustrates another symptom of addiction: *continued use despite the consequences.* Kipp had been warned repeatedly about what would happen, yet he persisted. In a sense, Kipp was very lucky: He got off with a light jail sentence and was ordered to enter a drug treatment program. But no matter how many warnings you give them, no matter how many horror stories you tell about the dangers of drugs, addicts just keep on snorting, smoking, and shooting up.

There's one more aspect of addiction that all drugs and alcohol abusers share in common: *denial.* Denial can even affect family members and friends by giving them reasons or excuses to not stand up and say enough is enough. Virtually none of my patients openly and freely admit they have a drug problem before they come in for treatment. They even use themselves as examples of sobriety or controlled use. It's much more common to hear patients say something like, "I don't have a problem. I can handle it. My parents (or my girlfriend or my bosses or my friends)—*they* have the problem." Yet the more evidence of their problem you put before them—lost jobs, broken relationships, illness—the more defensive they become.

Other Factors in Addiction

The emphasis of this chapter has been on the biological basis of addiction. As I've indicated, however, other factors are also important. It is entirely possible to develop an addictive disease in the absence of a biological predisposition. Or, as we've seen, addiction can result when predisposition succumbs to environmental pressure.

In this sense, addiction is no one's fault. Still, that doesn't mean addicts are off the hook in terms of responsibility. They may be born addicts, but that doesn't explain, nor does it excuse, their initial decision to use drugs. We may not be able to control our genetic structure, but we can control many of the environmental and life-style factors that lead to that fateful choice.

One of those factors is *attitude.* If you posses the attitude that drugs are bad, then you already are equipped with one of the strongest weapons against drugs. But if you live in a community or move in a social circle in which drug use is tolerated, or even approved, then you are at risk. Carla the Coed may have lived all her life in a small town where illicit drugs simply were not a part of the picture. Put her in a college dorm where everyone smokes pot every day, though, and the chances are she'll try it eventually.

And as I said, such experimental use will lead to tolerance, tolerance to abuse, and abuse to dependence.

From the sixties to the eighties our country's attitude toward drugs had been one of acceptance. We should take a warning from the experience of such countries as England and Sweden. Much to their chagrin, these nations, which have tolerated or legalized drugs, now find themselves swamped with addicts. For this and other reasons, I am vehemently opposed to legalization of drugs, a point I'll expand on in Chapter Twelve. Happily, though, as we move into the nineties, the American mood is shifting toward Zero Tolerance. Good news indeed.

Another factor in addiction is the sheer *availability* of a drug. One study showed that perhaps one in five American GIs stationed in Vietnam developed heroin addiction—Asia, after all, is prime real estate if you're a poppy grower. But 90 percent of those addicts gave up heroin once they returned to the United States, where they did not previously use the drug and where using it was difficult and not as rewarding. Drugs must be readily available and used with a specific set of expectations and in a specific setting. Most Vietnam addicts simply stopped when they were back home. Today, with drugs flooding our cities and with prices dropping, they are more widely available to more people than ever before.

Is there such a thing as an "addictive personality"? Not in my book. Nonetheless, some *personality traits,* such as immaturity, antisocial behavior, and high emotional dependency on others, may facilitate addiction. Peer influence or a disruption in someone's life—death of a loved one, relocation, career change—can also play a significant part.

A person's *occupation* may directly contribute to the use of drugs or even the choice of drugs. For example, at the turn of this century, one third of the cocaine and opiate addicts were health care professionals. While no definitive studies regarding the rate of alcoholism and addiction among today's health care professionals have been done, I would estimate that it exceeds the addiction rate for the general population (approximately 10 percent). Why are health care professionals, especially physicians and nurses, so prone to addiction?

First, there is *access.* Doctors and nurses have relatively easy access to a wide range of potentially addicting medications. Physicians have been known to "eat the mail" (consuming free samples of medications) and to self-prescribe medications for fake conditions.

Second, there is *familiarity.* Many physicians and nurses either prescribe or distribute powerful medications on a daily, even hourly, basis. Over time, this close association often dulls a physician's or nurse's wariness regarding these potentially addicting medications.

Third, there is *false security.* With a detailed knowledge of how the human body works, many physicians and nurses mistakenly assume that this knowledge gives them power over a drug, whether it is a prescription medication or an illicit drug. They assume they will be able to control a drug and stop before addiction occurs, since they think they know how a drug works as well as the signs of addiction. This assumption is just another example of how a drug user's denial can help them rationalize their drug taking. And addicted physicians and nurses often see their failure to control their addiction as a professional failing, something to be ashamed of, which often prevents them from seeking treatment.

Fourth, there is *ignorance.* The medical education of both physicians and nurses has often neglected the study of substance abuse and has impaired physicians and nurses in particular. By not giving these problems adequate attention, medical and nursing schools have contributed to substance abuse in our society and in their professions.

Fifth, there is *practice.* Doctors and nurses often experiment with drugs during training. Whether staying up late at night to study or to cope with working in the emergency room, or to get four hours of sleep after working 48 hours, drugs and alcohol are often taken as a means to help the students survive; when the drugs "work" they're taken again.

Add these five points to the life-and-death stress of a physician's or nurse's job and you have a prescription for addiction.

Fortunately, the situation is changing. Medical and nursing schools have increased their studies of addiction. Professional organizations, such as the American Medical Association and most state medical societies, have addressed the problem of impaired physicians and nurses through specialized identification, education, and treatment programs.

Still, you have to wonder why preemployment drug screening (with an application) is so strenuously avoided by medical schools! Why should a performer for an ABC soap opera have to be drug-free when a premed or medical student doesn't? I will never forget treating a young New York surgeon who told me he went into medicine "to get the best drugs." Certainly his was an unusual case, but the very real problem of impaired physicians should warrant the in-depth questioning and comprehensive drug testing of applicants *before* admission into medical school, internship, or residency.

In other professions, drug use and addiction have been more common because wealth and/or notoriety provided greater access to drugs and because drugs were viewed as symbols of success. These addicts of the late 1970s and early 1980s included rock stars, Wall Street traders, business leaders, movie idols and sports heroes. Not only have these VIPs been more likely to use drugs, but treating any subsequent addiction has been complicated by their wealth, status, and need for privacy. Often these VIP addicts demanded (and still demand) special treatment: private rooms, personal physicians, specially prepared food, and full-time assistants. Unfortunately, some treatment providers enhance the VIP patient's feelings of entitlement by treating them with awe—often with disastrous results. VIP patients have challenged the treatment system at all levels: from bringing their own physicians from the United Kingdom as "roommates," to having drugs delivered to the hospital in pizza cartons or flowers, to calling news conferences to announce their "cures."

In the 1970s, Fair Oaks in New Jersey treated a large number of celebrity heroin and/or cocaine addicts. We had so many of these celebrity patients that *Playboy* and a number of other publications profiled our program in the pre-Betty-Ford era. But before I could establish a celebrity treatment program, I had to institute an effective treatment program for all addicts. As a researcher and biological psychiatrist I had to answer a very basic question: How should I set up the *best* treatment program? Well, first I used my medical background and experience to evaluate addicts, find their medical problems, and treat them. Second, I used new treatments that we had pioneered to help detoxify the patients and keep them in treatment. Next, I mobilized the power of group therapy and added a 12 Step emphasis. Finally, we got the entire family and even the employer involved in the treatment process. Then the staff of nearly three professionals for every patient did the work.

We still had the problem of how to handle the rich and famous, i.e., the fly-in patient. My "celebrity" program at Fair Oaks was greatly influenced by New York Hospital expert and Cornell professor Bob Millman's concept of fighting the "entitlement" and creating a secure environment where names and "secrets" would be safe. As Dr. Millman explained, "To treat these patients you must focus on the *commonality* of addiction and not the differences between VIP patients and other patients." VIP patients should get the best treatment possible and not a new, untested, special "recipe"—to do so only encourages the addict's false sense of uniqueness ("That guy has a problem, but not me!") and interferes with successful treatment. Children of the rich and famous are sometimes the toughest VIP patients to treat. This group has learned the fruits and rewards of success but not how (or why) to be a success. Before treatment with this group can succeed, they must be taught how to live (habilitation) and not merely undergo drug rehabilitation.

We now know that addiction doesn't require any wealth,

prestige, or celebrity status to claim its victims; everyone from a CEO to a worker on a toaster-oven assembly line, is at risk. Workers may use drugs because they are bored, or because they think drugs give them more energy or make them more creative. Whatever the excuse, drugs have spread into the workplace at an alarming rate. The good news, though, is that many companies are sponsoring programs to help their employees get off drugs and stay off. Even better, more and more companies are implementing drug-prevention programs and drug-testing policies that prevent the problem from occurring in the first place. More on this important topic in Chapter Eleven.

One cause of addiction is the particular *actions of the drugs themselves.* As I'll describe in Chapter Seven, cocaine, especially in the form of crack, is frighteningly addictive, even to some people of the strongest genetic stock. A dangerous new drug known as "ice," a smokable form of amphetamine or "speed," acts in a similar way, as we'll see in Chapter Eight.

Some *environmental influences* can be very subtle. We now consider the mother's womb to be part of a person's environment. We know that maternal use of such drugs as alcohol, cocaine, "ice," and heroin can cause a baby to be born already addicted, or severely compromised. But it's possible, too, that a seemingly unrelated problem, like a reduction in the baby's oxygen supply during the process of birth, might trigger a process that could cause a disease gene to express itself. Even early parent-child reactions—too much or too little attention, or the wrong kind of nurturing—might do the same thing. In the not-too-distant future, we'll have a map that identifies all the genetic markers for psychiatric illnesses. With that to guide us, we can then look at other factors in the environment to see which ones may trigger the emergency of the disease.

Stress is another factor. Everyone suffers reversals in life—a promotion that doesn't come through, failure on the job or in relationships. Some people bounce back quickly and move on. But given enough stress applied at the right time and for sufficient duration, many people try to solve their problems with chemicals. Part of my work with patients involves showing them alternative ways of handling the stress that comes as a normal part of living.

Setting also makes a difference in the proclivity to use drugs and in the risks they pose. A person who wouldn't dream of using drugs in her parents' home might use heroin in Vietnam or rush back to her apartment after Sunday dinner to belt down a bottle of wine. For that matter, someone who gets plastered in his living room is much less of a danger to himself and others that if he were to get behind the wheel of a car.

People suffering from an *underlying disease* are more prone to substance abuse than others. Many use drugs as a means of coping with the pain of, say, cancer. Frequently, people will try to conceal or suppress their emotional problems, such as depression, through use of drugs or alcohol. But many people don't drink because they're depressed; they're depressed because they drink. As a doctor, my challenge is to sort out cause and effect. Interestingly, someone receiving morphine or heroin for pain will not become addicted or will only become addicted very slowly when compared to someone else who takes the same drug, in the same amount and frequency, to get high. I have to dig to discover whether the substance abuse is a problem at all. In cancer patients, the most common problem is the underprescription of pain medications.

Having given my definition of addiction and the factors that work together to produce addiction, let's take a look now at the addictive substances themselves.

CHAPTER FIVE

Alcohol: The Dazzle of the Devil

What other substance has come to symbolize the best and the worst of our culture? On the one hand, alcohol represents a central instrument in many of our most holy holidays, sacraments, and rituals, but to many others it stands for the devil's own drink. Clever marketing and advertising strategies have linked it with the lifestyles of the rich and famous, but a trip down our city streets reveals that it's also at home with poverty, homelessness, and destitution. Clearly, no substance has ever bedazzled and bedeviled to the same degree as alcohol.

I remember a conversation I had recently with an acquaintance of mine who, while lavishly extolling the virtues of a 1985 Bordeaux, suddenly joked, "But, of course, guys like you wouldn't understand."

Well, maybe he's right. As a physician, I see only the worst of alcohol: the addiction, the disease, and the deaths. If I could just snap my fingers and make alcohol disappear, I would do so without a moment's hesitation. But over many centuries alcohol has become such a fact of life that we are saddled with it. At least for the foreseeable future.

Fortunately, though, our society is seeing the light and is

changing its attitude about alcohol. Here are some items from the Good News file about our country:

- Use of alcohol is on the decline. From 1980 to 1987, beer consumption fell 7 percent and wine consumption 14 percent.
- Use of distilled spirits (gin, whiskey, and so on) is down a whopping 24 percent, to its lowest point in three decades.
- Leading hotel chains have stopped building or have removed their traditional liquor bars. As one executive stated, people today "don't want to be seen slugging down drinks like drunks."
- "Happy Hours," when drinks are foisted onto people at low prices, are becoming relics of the past.
- Deaths due to alcohol-related illness are decreasing; so too is the incidence of alcohol-related traffic deaths.
- Warning labels stating the dangers of drinking while pregnant now appear on all alcohol containers.
- More and more, people see that the use of alcohol is incompatible with a fit and healthy life-style.

As good as this news is, we have a long way to go. In this country, two out of three Americans still drink; half of those drink regularly—every day or a couple of times a week. Most of these people suffer no long-term ill effects from alcohol. But perhaps ten million Americans are problem drinkers—people whose use of alcohol creates psychological or social problems for themselves or others. Another ten million have the disease known as alcoholism and are addicted to alcohol. This is the group we call alcoholics. Alcohol remains the number-one drug of abuse for our children and teenagers. In the 1990 Partnership Study nearly 20 percent of all teens admitted that they have had five or more drinks at least once in the preceding two weeks.

Alcohol is a paradox. A small dose acts as a stimulant in some ways, a relaxant in others. But in only slightly higher doses alcohol reveals its true identity as a depressant and sedative.

Another paradox of alcohol is that it's a drink, but in some ways it's a food. Chock-full of calories—about 170 of them in an ounce—it provides the body with energy to burn. Cells in tissues use alcohol as they busily carry out their job of keeping us alive. But those calories are "empty"—alcohol has virtually no nutritive value, and contributes nothing to your recommended daily allowance of vitamins and minerals. Alcohol, like cocaine, interferes with appetite and destroys the taste for food. Problem drinkers ignore their need to eat, which leads to malnutrition.

Alcohol and Adolescents

At what age do people start drinking? Unfortunately, the age of first use gets lower every year. A 1989 survey conducted by PRIDE—the Parent's Resource Institute for Drug Education—found that 15 percent of kids in the sixth grade try alcohol. By the end of the ninth grade roughly half use liquor. By senior year, 70 percent of adolescents drink, and one out of 20 does so every day.

The number of teenage drinkers is about three-and-a-half times greater than the number of marijuana users and almost 20 times greater than cocaine users. In the 1990 Partnership Study approximately 29 percent of the teens surveyed reported a regular pattern of drinking. Even more frightening: Of the alcohol-drinking teens with a driver's license, 13 percent said that their ability to drive was impaired by alcohol at least once in the last 30 days!

I'm not surprised that so many kids drink. Our society sends them a very strong signal that booze is part of a happy, party-hearty life-style, confusing everyone to the extent that some young people come to believe that beer is not alcohol. Sports programs are saturated with ads featuring athletes touting their favorite brew. Rock concerts and television ads featuring rock stars are favorite venues for beer-company advertisements. Here's a shocker: By the time they graduate, high school seniors have been blasted by 100,000 TV ads for beer. That's not counting ads on the radio and in magazines, or ads for other alcohol products! The annual budget for promoting *one single brand of beer* in this country is $110 million—more than the entire national budget for alcohol research.

A recent survey turned up some other dismaying findings. For one thing, a lot of kids had no idea that those brightly colored, innocent looking "coolers," packaged and marketed like soda pop, contained wine! And guess which ads were rated among the favorites of high school boys—beer ads, of course, especially those featuring fast cars, rock stars, or Spuds MacKenzie, the "party animal" spokesdog for Budweiser.

If "Truth in Advertising" really existed, advertisers would use some sobering statistics and not cute animals to get their message across. Imagine advertisements proclaiming that alcohol-related highway accidents are the leading killer among people aged 15 to 24; drinking is the primary cause of traffic accidents among teenage drivers; about half of all youthful deaths in drowning, fires, suicide, and homicide are related in some way to alcohol use.

But a kid doesn't have to die to suffer from the effects of alcohol. Booze wrecks young bodies. Like any drug, alcohol interferes with emotional and physical development during the age when that development is reaching its peak. It disrupts social life and performance in school. A hangover passes after a few hours; some aftereffects of liquor, however, last a lifetime. Kids who drink are more likely to get in trouble with the law; girls are more likely to get pregnant.

Alcohol clouds judgments while increasing risk-taking behavior—a dangerous combination. One family whose son, a strapping, athletic, popular kid, got plastered one night, broke into the town swimming pool, and did a perfect half gainer into the water. Unfortunately, he didn't realize he was diving into the shallow end of the pool. He broke his neck and was completely paralyzed from the head down.

I was obviously elated when every state in the country raised its drinking age to 21. Now alcohol use by anyone younger than that is not just dangerous and stupid, it's illegal. This simple change has given parents another reason to say no to their kids. I'm still angry, though, that even with the drinking-age law on the books, some parents offer their friends' kids a drink or look the other way at their own parties.

I'm concerned because I know that early alcohol use could be the start of a lifetime of trouble with drugs. Kids who are predisposed to develop alcoholism become vulnerable as early as age 15. If they start drinking before then, it may be impossible to keep the illness from taking over their lives, or to treat them once it does.

Alcohol Opens Dangerous Doors

As firmly as any fact can be established, we know that alcohol and tobacco are gateway drugs. The term "gateway" means that once adolescents decide to use alcohol or cigarettes, they cross a threshold that makes it much easier to go on and use other drugs as well. The gateway concept was ridiculed in the sixties by people—some of them experts—who glibly pointed out that "100 percent of marijuana smokers started out drinking milk, so milk must also be a 'gateway' drug."

Well, we may not have had the facts then, but we've got them now. Research shows clearly that a kid who drinks liquor at 16 is three times as likely to become a heavy drinker as an adult than someone who doesn't use alcohol until after the age of 21. A study by PRIDE found that more than half of the high school seniors who use cocaine began drinking beer and smoking cigarettes at age 13 or under. A third of them began their involvement with alcohol and tobacco before the age of 11!

In those vulnerable years, kids who learn to rely on chemicals to get through troubled times may need that crutch for the rest of their lives. The longer we can delay a person's decision to use drugs, the better the odds are that the person will never become chemically dependent. Curbing early use of tobacco and alcohol would go a long way in preventing future use of cocaine, marijuana, and other substances of abuse.

Alcohol: What It Is and What it Does

The "active ingredient" in alcoholic beverages is ethyl alcohol (ethanol). We get ethanol by mixing yeast with foods high in sugary carbohydrates. The yeast secretes an enzyme that breaks the sugar into carbon dioxide and alcohol—the process known as fermentation. When the alcohol concentration gets too high (around 14 percent), the yeast dies, thus stopping natural fermentation. Distilling is a way of artificially boosting the alcohol content of liquors such as whiskey. The alcohol in a product is expressed in terms of "proof"; the proof value is double the percentage of alcohol. Thus 80-proof scotch, for example, is 40 percent pure alcohol.

About 20 percent of the alcohol you drink is immediately absorbed from the stomach into the bloodstream. The rest passes into the small intestine and is then absorbed. Because alcohol is a relatively small and simple molecule, it can go just about anywhere in the body it wants to. One place it loves to hang out is the brain. Usually the brain is protected from chemical attack by a membrane that filters out any suspiciously large or threatening substances. Alcohol, however, squeezes through this membrane and, like a monkey in the cockpit, starts screwing around with the electrical and chemical switches it finds.

Your body, though, works to eliminate alcohol as fast as it can. One way it does so is through the breath, which is why Breathalyzer tests can reveal the level of intoxication. Mostly, though, it's the liver that does the hard work. The liver secretes a succession of enzymes, which clip off parts of the alcohol molecule and send them on their way. Depending on your size, weight, and metabolism, your body can usually keep up with you if you drink about one ounce of whiskey or three ounces of wine in an hour. More than that, however, alcohol builds up, as do its intoxicating effects.

For the record, those effects include increased heart rate, flushing, and loss of alertness. As the amount rises, your perception is altered, your vision is blurred, and your coordination falls apart. In other words, you get drunk. Interestingly, the word "intoxicated" means "shot with a poisoned arrow"—a fitting description.

The Physical Consequences of Alcohol

The "poison arrow" of intoxication has many long-term effects. Unfortunately, many alcoholics suffering from these effects never receive proper treatment or evaluation. Usually, the patients will be treated for an alcohol-related condition, pancreatitis, for example, without the physician ever probing for signs of alcohol abuse. The doctor may ask a few questions about drinking or drug use, but frequently they'll accept the patient's answers at face value (even though alcoholics, like all addicts, are notorious liars). On other occasions, the substance abuse will be identified, but underlying conditions such as a nutritional imbalance will go untreated.

In this section, I'll discuss the major areas of the body that bear the brunt of chronic alcohol abuse and the many subsequent physical problems that may force an alcoholic to seek help.

Liver Disease Show me a heavy drinker, and I'll show you a damaged liver. Liver damage from alcohol consumption falls into three categories: (1) fatty liver; (2) alcoholic hepatitis; (3) cirrhosis. At one time, it was thought that these conditions were progressive; now we know that cirrhosis can occur without a history of hepatitis. The incidence of these conditions among heavy drinkers is startling: close to 100 percent have fatty livers, 10 to 35 percent get alcoholic hepatitis, while 10 to 20 percent will eventually develop cirrhosis (this estimate may be low, since autopsies suggest that 40 percent of all cases of cirrhosis go undetected.) The good news is that both fatty liver and hepatitis can be reversed with abstinence from alcohol. Unfortunately, abstinence does not reverse cirrhosis.

Fatty deposits enlarge and cause oxygen depletion in the liver, a factor that may cause alcoholic liver disease. Hepatitis is a viral infection of the liver that can lead to cirrhosis, a disease in which liver cells are progressively destroyed and replaced by nodules that are largely scar tissue. Each year, cirrhosis ranks among the top ten killers in America.

How much alcohol consumption is necessary to cause liver damage? Increased risk of fatty liver deposits have been associated with as little as six drinks a day for men and only one to two drinks daily for women! Cirrhosis will usually develop given enough time and enough alcohol (drinking a little more than two sixpacks a day for 20 years has been associated with a 50 percent incidence of cirrhosis).

Gastrointestinal Disorders Alcohol and ulcers go hand-in-hand. In the past, science believed that little alcohol was metabolized in the stomach. Recently, it has been established that a significant percentage of low doses of alcohol (so-called social drinking) is broken down in the stomach. Alcohol has a nasty effect on the stomach for two reasons. First, the stomach is exposed to more alcohol than virtually any other part of the body. Second, alcohol seems to interfere with the protective mucus that lines the stomach, leading to the spread of gastric acids into the stomach lining.

Heavy alcohol consumption is a leading factor behind another painful gastrointestinal disorder, pancreatitis. Pancreatitis is the inflammation of the pancreas, a gland located behind the stomach that is responsible for secreting insulin and other hormones involved in the metabolism of sugar. Exactly what causes pancreatitis isn't known, but some researchers believe that digestive enzymes that normally work outside the pancreas get "switched on" inside the pancreas. Alcohol is thought to reduce levels of substances within the pancreas that are responsible for keeping these digestive enzymes under wraps. Pancreatitis is characterized by severe abdominal pain, nausea, vomiting, and rapid heartbeats.

Most patients respond within a few days to standard treatments of intravenous fluids and painkillers. However, about 20 percent of patients develop a chronic and more severe form of the disease; in rare cases it may be fatal.

Nutritional Disorders A whole host of nutritional disorders are associated with heavy alcohol consumption. These disorders include malnutrition, anemia, neuropathy (the disruption of the peripheral nervous system), and even osteoporosis. While a poor diet is believed to be primarily responsible for these deficiencies, there is additional evidence that alcohol itself interferes with the normal metabolism of food.

Heart Disease Cardiac disease, along with liver disease, is one of the major reasons for the high death rate among alcoholics. While some recent reports have trumpeted the positive effects of low alcohol consumption on the heart, heavy drinking has a clearly negative effect. Alcohol attacks the heart on several fronts: it weakens the heart muscle (cardiomyopathy), it may lead to high blood pressure (hypertension), and it may be responsible for reduced blood flow in the heart (ischemic heart disease).

Exactly why alcohol leads to cardiomyopathy—the number one cause of heart transplants—is not known, but some researchers believe that it reduces the breakdown of fatty acids in the heart (also increasing triglyceride content) and interferes with mitochondria (the tiny energy-producing structures in the heart.) Both of these actions may lead directly to alcohol-induced cardiomyopathy.

Besides alcohol's direct attack upon the heart muscle, alcohol has also been associated with another leading factor in heart disease, hypertension. One study found that people who had six or more drinks a day were twice as likely to suffer from high blood pressure when compared to nondrinkers or moderate drinkers (two or less drinks daily). It has also been found that a single drink will cause the release of hormones that will ultimately raise a person's blood pressure.

Fetal Alcohol Syndrome One of the most disturbing physical effects of alcohol is its physical effect upon the fetus. In 1973, after centuries of alcohol consumption during pregnancy, medical science finally established a direct link between alcohol and a pattern of birth defects. In 1988, more than $300 million was spent in the treatment of these birth defects. Each year, as many as three babies out of every 1,000 births are estimated to be born suffering from alcohol-induced birth defects.

Recently, one large-scale study found that 84 percent of people aged 18 to 44 were vaguely aware of the dangers of drinking during pregnancy, but only a fraction of them understood that drinking during pregnancy can cause birth defects. In fact, a majority of respondents mistakenly associated FAS with alcohol addiction in the newborn. Actually, the following conditions are associated with drinking during pregnancy:

1. Distorted facial appearance.
2. Mental retardation or other forms of central nervous system dysfunction.
3. Decreased birth weight.

Alone, each of the above conditions is classified as a fetal alcohol effect (FAE); when combined they qualify as fetal alcohol syndrome (FAS).

Even drinking as little as one ounce of alcohol a day (the equivalent of one beer) has been associated with lower birth weights and spontaneous abortions. However, in general, the risk of alcohol consumption and subsequent birth defects follows a continuum: The more alcohol consumed, the greater the risk of FAS or FAE.

While much is known about FAS after a baby is born, very little is known about the effects of alcohol on the fetus. Animal studies have pointed to several possible explanations for FAS.

First, alcohol consumption during pregnancy has been found to result in decreased fetal activity and shorter umbilical cords. Decreased fetal activity and short umbilical cords are factors that have been associated with physical defects and growth retardation.

Second, alcohol consumption adversely affects the fetus's ability to regulate its body temperature, greatly endangering the baby's health.

Third, prenatal alcohol exposure has been associated with an increased response to stress. In humans, one way we have of measuring our response to stress is to monitor the activity of the hypothalamic, pituitary, and adrenal glands (called the HPA axis) and the subsequent levels of corticosteroids produced by the HPA axis. The more stress affects us, the greater the activity of HPA axis and the levels of corticosteroids in the blood. Animals exposed to alcohol in the fetus have shown an elevated stress response when compared to animals that were not exposed to alcohol. In humans, this may result in babies that are abnormally bothered by even the slightest movements, noises, or changes in the environment.

Fourth, brain activity in animals has been shown to be affected in numerous ways by alcohol exposure during pregnancy. For example, fetal alcohol exposure reduced the overall weight of the brain, especially in the hippocampus, an area of the brain involved in the stress response. Other areas of the brain responsible for central nervous system development were also adversely effected by alcohol.

Children born with FAS face a difficult future. Almost all will require specialized educational training. Studies have found that FAS children can make impressive strides in improving their concentration, coordination, and behavior. However, when compared to normal children, FAS children had higher rates of psychological disorders and learning disabilities (such as hyperactivity, anxiety, and speech disability).

One final note: When experts call for legalization of drugs, I can't help but think of the hundreds of years—and of the countless numbers of babies born with birth defects—that passed before the recognition of FAS. If we legalize drugs, how many years and how many babies will it take to recognize Fetal Cocaine Syndrome or Fetal Marijuana Syndrome?

Alcoholism

No discussion of the physical disorders caused by alcohol would be complete without a thorough discussion of *alcoholism.* Alcoholism is a physical disease that renders its victims highly susceptible to the effects of ethanol. Alcoholics—a better term is "people with alcoholism"—are drinkers whose use of alcohol has proceeded through the stages of use/tolerance/dependency/abuse until they have become addicted, both physically and psychologically. For a list of definitions of terms, see Box on page 99.

Alcohol produces dependence as surely as will any other central nervous system depressant, such as barbiturates. Dependency is the first sign that the heavy drinker has a problem that has spiraled out of control.

Alcoholism shares the classic features of other addictions: preoccupation with getting the drug, compulsive use, relapse, and denial. Once the disease has reached this point (but preferably long before), the alcoholic needs immediate professional help. I'll have much more to say about that topic in later chapters.

As I explained in Chapter Four, alcoholism is a physical illness that to a large extent arises from biological traits passed on from parent to child. In fact, a family history of alcoholism is the biggest risk factor for developing the disease. The odds of sharing the trait of alcoholism are as high as the odds of developing ulcers or diabetes—two other illnesses known to be handed down through the generations. In my experience, perhaps half the people with alcoholism have a family history of the disease. If we define *familial alcoholism* as a major problem with alcohol among first-degree relatives (parents and siblings) or second-degree relatives (grandparents, aunts and uncles, and so on), then as many as 80 percent of the alcoholics entering treatment could be said to have a familial form of the disorder.

Researchers have identified two distinct types of alcoholism, each with its own syndrome, or pattern of symptoms. What we call *Type 1* alcoholism is commonly seen in people who are related to *female* alcoholics. The disease usually develops after the age of 25. People with this alcoholic syndrome can refrain from drinking alcohol for periods of time and seldom get into fights or get arrested for drunk driving. However, they quickly

Alcohol Abuse: Some Definitions

Alcoholism: A chronic primary hereditary disease that progresses from an early, physiological susceptibility into an addiction characterized by tolerance changes, physiological dependence, and loss of control over drinking. Psychological symptoms are secondary to the physiological disease and not relevant to its onset.

Recovery: A return to normal functioning based on total, continuous abstinence from alcohol and substitute drugs, corrective nutrition, and an accurate understanding of the disease.

Problem drinker: A person who is not an alcoholic but whose alcohol use creates psychological and social problems for himself and/or others.

Heavy drinker: Anyone who drinks frequently or in large amounts. A heavy drinker may be a problem drinker, an alcoholic, or a normal drinker with a high tolerance for alcohol.

Alcoholic: A person with the disease of alcoholism.

(Adapted from James R. Milam and Katherine Ketcham. *Under the Influence: A Guide to the Myths and Realities of Alcoholism,* New York: Bantam Books, 1983, p. 189. Used by permission.)

develop a severe psychological dependence on alcohol and have trouble controlling or stopping a binge once it starts. They suffer from guilt and fear about their dependence and have a high rate of liver complications. Type 1 alcoholics are passive and dependent people, with a low need for novelty and a high need to avoid harm. These people tend to use alcohol because it relieves their anxiety.

Type 2 alcoholism is more often seen in people related to *male* alcoholics. Type 2 alcoholics, mostly men, usually develop the illness before age 25. They find it difficult to abstain from drinking, are more likely to get into fights and to be arrested for reckless driving while drinking, and are more likely to be treated for alcohol abuse at some point. This group tends to have antisocial personalities and to use alcohol for the feeling of euphoria it supplies, rather than to relieve anxiety.

Type 1 alcoholism is more common and affects both men and women. Although there is a strong genetic basis for this illness, its severity and onset are affected by the person's environment. Type 2 alcoholism, seen in about one out of four male alcoholics, is almost entirely genetic; environment has very little to do with triggering this illness.

As I've stated, one way to distinguish between the types of alcoholism is by the age at which the illness develops. As many as 86 percent of patients whose alcoholism emerged early (around age 16) have a family history of alcoholism. Even among those who didn't become alcoholics until past the age of 40, 41 percent reported alcoholism in the family.

Alcoholism can be passed on directly from parent to child. But alcoholism can also emerge as a trait in families who suffer from other psychiatric disorders. Researchers have found alcoholism is very common in male relatives of women with mood disorders such as depression. The reverse is also true: mood disorders often crop up in female relatives of alcoholic men.

Depression isn't the only psychiatric disorder involved. Alcoholism is also more common in families with anxiety disorders (particularly panic disorders), eating disorders, and agoraphobia (fear of leaving the home).

Surveys also reveal a higher rate of alcoholism among relatives of cocaine and other drug abusers, even those who do not also abuse alcohol, than is found in the general population. And there is a higher incidence of drug dependence among relatives of alcoholics, even those alcoholics who do not also abuse drugs.

Such results suggest that in some families alcoholism and drug abuse is part of a spectrum of mood disorders and other psychiatric problems with a powerful genetic component. There may turn out to be a "substance abuse gene" or sequence of genes. In 1990, researchers at the University of Texas reported that they may have found the genetic link to alcoholism. This gene, called the dopamine D2 receptor gene, was present in 69 percent of the severe alcoholics that were studied, but in only 20 percent of the nonalcoholics (other researchers, however, have failed to confirm this finding.) Depending on a person's gender, environment, and development, those genes might express themselves as an addiction to cocaine or alcohol, a mood disorder, or some combination of these.

When it comes to heredity, some genes never have a chance. In other words, without the proper environment, or without a triggering event at the right moment, the trait encoded in that gene may never express itself in a person's body or behavior. Studies indicate that three out of four cases of alcoholism result from some mix of biogenetic, psychosocial, and environmental influences.

We know that, for some women, their substance abuse problem results from the behavior of important people in their lives. Many of our women patients tell me they only drink or use drugs when married to or living with a substance abuser. In treatment we help these women disengage from another person's illness so they don't get dragged down themselves.

These genetic and environmental studies are part of the good news because they increase our understanding of alcoholism enormously. More important, they have real bearing on how we attack the problem. Because Type 2 alcoholics, for example, are almost predestined to express the illness, their treatment should focus on ways to manage a chronic disease. Type 1 alcoholics may benefit more from strategies designed to prevent the onset of the disease and to relieve guilt and anxiety with psychotherapy and medications.

In addition to genetic inheritance, other physical traits can contribute to the emergence of alcoholism. For example, in 1983 scientists discovered that alcoholics have higher levels of an enzyme that helps the body cope with the toxic effect of alcohol. Normally, people have a limited amount of this enzyme. When they drink too much, the enzyme is overwhelmed and can't break down the alcohol fast enough. Thus people feel sick, an event that tends to make them prefer to drink less. A low enzyme level thus defends against indulgence. With their higher enzyme levels, however, alcoholics can drink more without feeling bad. This explains why, in the earlier stages of their illness at least, many alcoholics seem better able to "hold their liquor" than the average Joe.

Brain-wave readings on alcoholics reveal abnormalities in those parts of the brain associated with memory and emotion. These odd readings persist, even in alcoholics who no longer drink. For that matter, about 40 percent of the children of alcoholics also show this unusual brain-wave pattern—more evidence that heredity is a factor in the disease. We don't yet know how, or even whether, these brain patterns contribute to the onset or severity of alcoholism. But they do provide more evidence that people who are susceptible to alcohol are physically different in some ways.

Other studies showed that the brain of a person susceptible to alcohol may transmit messages at a slightly slower rate than in normal people. This delayed rate does not affect a person's intelligence, but it may cause people at risk to be less willing or able to pay as much attention to their surroundings—a classic symptom of attention-deficit hyperactivity disorder (ADHD) and of antisocial personality disorder. Such findings suggest that a person born with even minimum brain dysfunction may be more vulnerable to alcoholism.

Recently some investigators reported the results of a study in which nine out of twelve men with a family history of alcoholism felt euphoric—"high"—after taking an antianxiety medication called alprazolam (sold under the name Xanax). Such a finding suggests that alcoholics are highly sensitive to this drug and perhaps others in its class (the benzodiazepines, including diazepam, better known as Valium). They may be at high risk for abusing such medications.

In addition to these short-term effects, regular use of alcohol can lead to feelings of sadness or anxiety, hyperactivity, and irritability. Chronic heavy use may cause such pyschiatric symptoms as paranoia, hallucinations, and insomnia.

Psychiatric Disorders That Resemble Alcoholism

Earlier I described Type 1 and Type 2 alcoholism. Actually, both of these types are considered to be *primary alcoholism,* in which alcohol abuse is the *cause of the problem.* The majority of alcoholics suffer from primary alcoholism.

Secondary alcoholism, in contrast, arises as the *result of some other problem,* such as a disease or a psychological disorder. A small but significant percentage of my patients who abuse alcohol do so not so much because they are biologically vulnerable, but as a response to some other severe illness, such as clinical depression.

This key distinction is crucial when it comes to helping people get better. It's a frustratingly typical scenario: Patients go to psychiatrists for help with their depression and anxiety. During an interview the doctor asks, "Do you use alcohol?" "Oh yes," the occasionally honest patient replies, "I drink every night." At that point the doctor needs to hear nothing more. She usually evaluates the person medically for the many problems that can be caused by alcohol and treats those that can be found. Often she calls for a family meeting and suggests that the family and the alcoholic attend Al-Anon and AA meetings, and that's that. What is difficult to pick up is that her patient's depression may not always stem from his drinking; the drinking can actually arise from the depression in certain cases! Unless she realizes that, and follows the patient's response to alcoholism treatment, she probably won't get to treat the *real* problem, and the patient will not improve completely.

Are doctors too eager to blame alcohol for all of the patients' problems? Not really. In the past, some of my fellow physicians dragged their heels when it came to naming "alcoholism" as the primary diagnosis. The stigma associated with that word is still very strong today, even in our supposedly enlightened age. Many people would rather be seen as having depression or even a personality disorder than be labeled an "alcoholic." This is especially the case with women. Although the situation is changing, many mental health professionals still seem blind to the fact that their female patients may be alcohol abusers. They tend to see their problem as one of anxiety or depression, and thus tend to underprescribe AA and overprescribe medications for these conditions. As I've mentioned, not only do these pills fail to attack the underlying problem, they pose a great risk of abuse, including overdosing or addiction. Such doctors risk becoming "enablers"—unwitting accomplices to the crime of substance abuse.

The problem of misdiagnosis (and thus mistreatment) is complicated by the fact that so many patients abuse alcohol, and that so many alcoholics have some other illness. Let's look at some of the common "mimickers"—the psychiatric and physical disorders that often get tangled up with the problem of alcoholism.

Depression As many as 60 percent of alcoholics may also suffer from depression. If there are ten million alcoholics in this country—a conservative estimate—then there are perhaps six million alcoholics with depression. It's not clear, though, how many of these people have depression induced by alcohol (the vast majority), and how many are simply self-medicating their preexisting depression by drinking.

A great many alcoholics with major depression are not being treated for their mood disorder. Some of these people, of course, simply do not see any doctors at all. Others may not have their true mood disorder identified since alcoholism and depression share a number of symptoms in common: insomnia, loss of appetite, depressed mood, guilty thoughts, loss of energy, and reduced interest in sex. Even the well-trained eye, then, may have trouble distinguishing one disorder from the other. One way to do so is to have the patient admitted to a hospital so he or she can "dry out." We have always felt that any symptoms that remain after 28 days of complete abstinence and active 12 Step treatment are probably due to the depression and not to the use of alcohol.

One of biopsychiatry's most important contributions is to

use laboratory testing to confirm a diagnosis, identify complications, and suggest avenues for treatment. Drug and alcohol testing from blood and urine samples, along with HIV (AIDS) testing, vitamin deficiency tests, and certain neuroendocrine tests that measure the levels and actions of certain hormones and steroids, for example, can give us a vivid picture of what's really happening inside the patient's body. These tests, together with careful psychiatric evaluation after detoxification and 28 days of abstinence and treatment, usually allow us to identify the alcoholic patient who also has a major depressive illness or some other physical disorder.

Overuse of alcohol can also cause elevations in a steroid called cortisol. Too much cortisol leads to a condition known as Cushing's syndrome, with its symptoms of moon-shaped face, mental or emotional disturbances, high blood pressure, weight gain, and, in women, abnormal growth of facial and body hair. Following cortisol levels can tell us whether these symptoms are truly a problem with cortisol secretion or whether they are transient and will abate when drinking ceases.

Malnutrition and diseases of the liver or pancreas (see above) can also produce symptoms mimicking depression. Patients with alcoholic cirrhosis of the liver have abnormal levels of a chemical known as butanediol. A test showing the presence of this chemical acts as a red flag, warning that the patient may be at risk. If cirrhosis is caught early enough, treatment can prevent loss of the liver and death. My job as a physician is to look for those problems and rule them out through an interview, examination, and careful lab testing before deciding on a course of treatment. Careful evaluation may also reveal a specific vitamin deficiency that may be contributing to the patient's depression.

Panic and Anxiety Most alcoholics complain of anxiety and many use alcohol in a vain attempt to cope with these feelings. Some, however, have a full-fledged panic disorder, marked by incapacitating panic attacks and anticipatory anxiety. Many of my patients mention that, in the early stage of their illness, they used alcohol to fend off these attacks. Unfortunately, they then became addicted to alcohol, and needed higher and more frequent doses of booze to ward off panic. Some patients develop panic attacks after they become dependent on alcohol. Other patients have panic attacks or "dry drunks" (panic, and irrational or agitated behavior and/or thoughts that mimic the person's actions while drunk) for months after complete abtinence.

Panic attacks—a medically recognized disorder—are characterized by palpitations, sweating, chest or abdominal pain, fear of impending doom, flushing, and tremor. Since this also describes the symptoms of alcohol withdrawal, doctors must take care to rule out the presence of a panic disorder. It's also important to rule out medical conditions that can mimic panic disorder, including low blood sugar, hyperthyroidism, and a heart condition known as mitral valve prolapse, which we have found in many alcoholics with panic disorder and which can respond to the use of certain cardiac medications. Withdrawal from opiates, barbiturates, or anxiety drugs can also produce symptoms of panic. Again, letting a patient dry out will help reveal which symptoms are related to use of alcohol and which are part of some other medical problem. However, whether the symptoms reflect true panic or alcoholism remains a very difficult diagnosis.

Schizophrenia The psychotic symptoms of alcohol intoxication or withdrawal can resemble the psychosis seen in people with schizophrenia. But only a few alcoholic patients actually suffer from schizophrenia. Psychosis induced by drink usually vanishes a few days after drinking stops. If it persists, the patient may have some kind of organic brain disorder, which brain scans and other tests can reveal.

Mania Some alcoholic patients experience sudden manic episodes marked by elation, hyperactivity, agitation, and rapid thoughts and speech. The first step is to determine whether this patient has delirium tremens—the DTs. Properly treated, patients with the DTs usually calm down quickly. Alcohol withdrawal can also mimic an acute manic episode. Hallucinations or paranoia are sometimes present; if these symptoms stem from the use of alcohol, they can be treated more easily and will subside more quickly than if they stem from a true case of mania. Many alcoholic patients abuse other substances, including cocaine, amphetamines, and hallucinogens, which can also produce symptoms that mimic mania. Such symptoms tend to vanish quickly if the problem is something other than a manic disorder.

Personality Disorders An alcoholic may have some kind of personality disorder, such as: borderline (having problems with identity, anger, unstable moods); narcissistic (self-important, prone to fantasies of limitless success, need for constant attention), or histrionic (excitable, overreactive, attention-seeking). Studies show that an alcoholic male is four times more likely to have an antisocial personality disorder than a nonalcoholic male; for women with alcoholism, the rate is 12 times as high. A physician who is aware of these cross-complications will know how to tease the symptoms of one apart from the symptoms of the other, and will treat the patient accordingly. When both the 12 Step and biopsychiatric treatment are firmly established, calling upon a therapist or psychoanalyst to help modify the personality disorders is next.

Dual Diagnosis Many times a patient seems to have one psychiatric illness but turns out to have another, or more than one. However, it is of course possible for a patient to have one or more than one medical or psychiatric condition at the same time. The problem, known as dual diagnosis, is a constant challenge.

Perhaps half of the patients in a typical doctor's practice have significant medical and psychosocial problems associated with alcohol abuse. Reports indicate that 22 percent of pati admitted for the treatment of substance abuse also met the criteria for bipolar mood disorder. Others have signs of attention-deficit hyperactivity disorder. Up to half of the cocaine addicts I treat also meet the criteria for major depression after they have been weaned from their drug.

The chances of successful therapy improve if the doctor can identify the patient's specific problems and choose the right treatment for each of them. Fortunately, treatment for substance abuse often does a great deal to improve the patient's other psychiatric conditions.

Children of Alcoholics

The children of alcoholics are at high risk of developing the illness themselves. But even if they never touch a drop, their lives can be hell because of the impact of the disease on their families. Fights, parental absences, illness, money troubles, ruined careers—all of these can scar the child from an alcoholic family. The scars persist into adulthood, causing pain and trouble long after the alcoholic parent is dead and buried.

Children of alcoholics, or COAs, can be any age. (Older ones are often called adult children of alcoholics, or ACOAs.) Regardless of age, they need help, and fortunately that help exists. Part of the good news in the treatment of alcoholism today is the focus on the needs of COAs. The COA movement has become a national phenomenon.

Awareness of the problem of COAs has led to an understanding of the suffering these people go through. Children of alcoholics tend to become "superchildren," taking on the responsibility of running the family, feeding their parents, and hiding the truth from the world. They love and fear their parents. But they don't realize they can't "save" their parents from their own destruction and thus feel horribly guilty over their constant failure. They are often abused, verbally if not physically. They thus have very poor self-images and low self-esteem, and they may find it impossible to develop satisfactory relationships with others outside the home. They grow to mistrust all people, but ironically come to tolerate intolerable behavior. Sometimes it's this clash of feelings that triggers the onset of their own alcoholism.

Even if these children do not turn into alcoholics, they often suffer psychological problems. Such problems may emerge as an obsessive-compulsive disorder—excessive concern about cleanliness, for example—or in a debilitating need to be 100 percent perfect all the time. Through their constant search for approval from others, and by always placing other people's needs ahead of their own, adult children of alcoholics get used to living with people who can't function. Often one result is that they fall into the trap of forming similar relationships, known as "codependent" relationships.

Codependency—the well-deserved hot topic of the talk-show circuit and the best-seller lists—means an unhealthy attachment to someone who has basically stopped functioning as a human being due to drinking, drugs, or other mental problems. Adult children of alcoholics may find themselves unable to confront their spouse's or child's drinking or drug problem directly. Instead, they do what they have always done: They try to control the other person's problems indirectly. They continue to lie, cover up, and clean up after the alcoholic, thinking that they do so out of love. Sometimes they harbor secret fantasies that through their loving patience, through their constant devotion, they will somehow cure their loved ones of their disease.

Without realizing it, though, they begin to define their whole identity in terms of their loved one's substance abuse problem. The dutiful wife or husband sees the spouse's problem as his or her cross to bear in life. In fact, if you were to wave a magic wand and cure the substance abuse problem forever, the codependent person would be shattered. Without a drunk to look after, the codependent has no identity, no task in life, no reason for living!

Redefining the problem of substance abuse in terms of the family—even in terms of generations—has opened many people's eyes. As we'll see in Chapter Sixteen, we've made tremendous strides in designing treatment that addresses the needs, not just of substance abusers themselves, but of the entire family. When everyone around the alcohol or drug addict understands their role in treatment, the chances of success rise astronomically.

CHAPTER SIX

Marijuana: The Illusion of Smoke

Bryce was 14 when he smoked his first joint.

"My best friend at the time was this guy who always had pot," recalled Bryce, who, at age 27, had come to Fair Oaks Hospital seeking help for his drug problem. "He kept pushing it on me. I tried it, but it didn't do anything for me. I remember thinking, 'So what's the big deal?' My friend said 'You gotta get used to it.' I told him it was a waste, that I couldn't get high. But I knew my friend wouldn't want to hang around with me anymore unless I smoked. So I did. At first I sort of faked like I was high, you know? But the third or fourth time, I didn't have to fake it. It hit me—and I felt great.

"For a while I smoked every day after school. Then one semester my first class of the day was math. I couldn't handle that. I started toking up on the way to school so I could get through math class without losing my mind. I kept getting okay grades—mostly Bs, a few Cs—so I figured pot wasn't hurting anything."

Over the course of a year or so, Bryce found that drugs became the focus of his world. "I quit the swim team—who needed that hassle? It was more fun to go to someone's house and get blasted and watch TV. Pretty soon we got into some of the hard stuff—LSD was our big thing. I'd tell my parents I was going on a trip for the weekend and they'd say, 'Bye, have a nice time.' They didn't know I was over at a friend's house on the next block fried to the eyeballs."

Bryce didn't date much. "Most of the girls weren't into drugs. I went out with somebody for a while, but she kept trying to get me to quit pot. I didn't need that kind of hassle, so I dumped her."

He graduated, but just barely. His grades weren't good enough to get him into the college he wanted. "I took courses at a technical school, but one day I thought, 'Jeez, I guess I don't really want to repair toasters for the rest of my life.' "

For years Bryce bounced from job to job, moving to different cities, losing contact with his family and former friends. Wherever he went, though, he quickly found a circle of drug users to hang out with. "I discovered that, if you got an ounce of pot or a gram of coke, you've always got lots of friends."

For the past year, however, Bryce had been vaguely aware of an emptiness at the center of his life. The feeling eventually became overpowering. He suffered from a bad bout of depression. "Some people I knew said I must have scored some bad dope. But even when I quit drugs for a while, that feeling was still there. I just wanted to die."

Bryce had been at Fair Oaks for about a week, undergoing intensive psychiatric evaluation. During one of our private counseling sessions, Bryce said, with sudden and surprising insight: "I'm 27 years old, and I don't know who I am or what I want."

We spent much of the rest of his therapy exploring this idea. Bryce realized how, by falling into drugs at such a vulnerable age, he had avoided the need to develop a sense of his own identity. With drugs as his anchor, he had never left port. He formed no lasting bonds with other people; the friendships he struck up were drug-induced illusions that vanished when the drugs ran out. He had built no career for himself, disguising his fear of making choices in a neverending search to stay high.

Bryce had failed to accomplish the basic tasks of growing up: to leave indulgence and fantasy behind, to discover and explore his own identity, and to move forward with confidence into the real world.

Adolescence is the worst possible time to use drugs—the adolescent who does may kill his chances for a happy adulthood. The maturing body has a lot of work to do switching on the machinery of sexual development; the last thing it needs is to be doused with poisons that disrupt the secretion of hormones and interfere with growth. And the maturing mind lacks the foresight and perspective necessary to question the wisdom of using drugs and to assess the evidence of risk.

The teen years are troubling enough. The pressure on kids is enormous: They are learning to separate from their families, to form relationships with members of the opposite sex, to make decisions about careers that will affect the rest of their lives. Bring pot into the picture, and you wind up with kids who "zonk out" and ignore their responsibilities to themselves or who chase grandiose and ultimately futile fantasies. In short, you wind up with Bryce—a perpetual adolescent, with no goals or direction. The psychoanalyst Erik Erikson has shown that the failure to master a developmental stage results in the failure to master subsequent developmental stages.

If alcohol is our most abused legal drug, marijuana is our most widely abused *illegal* drug. Four out of ten Americans have smoked pot at least once. A $10-billion-a-year industry, marijuana is the third biggest cash crop in the country; in some states—California, for example—it's actually number one. We grow more marijuana than soybeans, grapes, lettuce, and tomatoes. In fact, the Drug Enforcement Administration predicts that America will soon be—if it isn't already—the largest pot producer in the world.

For decades, controversy has swirled around the issue of just how dangerous marijuana is. The government-sponsored campaign of the 1930s tried to whip up anti-pot hysteria by exaggerating its effects. By the 1960s, though, users defended marijuana as being no more dangerous than an after-dinner drink. Since then an entire generation has grown up believing that marijuana is risk free. The truth, of course, lies somewhere in between.

The debate over the safety of marijuana too often runs aground because *both* sides have lacked the facts they need to make their case. Those who try to point out the drug's dangers often cite a few anecdotes and claim, wrongly, that such anecdotes constitute proof. They cite the conclusions of studies that were not done under rigorous scientific standards or that have long since been discredited. Their basic message is correct—pot is dangerous—but their proof is flimsy.

Promarijuana people then seize on these weaknesses in the data and claim, equally wrongly, that the *lack* of evidence is, in itself, proof of marijuana's safety.

Ironically, they have a point; we know far less about marijuana than we do about most prescription medications, which, because they have proven therapeutic value, have been studied thoroughly under controlled conditions in well-defined groups of people. We even know more about narcotics, whose chemical properties are simple and whose effects are relatively straightforward.

The good news is that the situation is changing. We realize now that earlier research was done on marijuana that was perhaps 30 times less potent than the pot available today. Because the new high-power strains have been around long enough, we are now accumulating hard evidence that dope does cause long-term physical, psychological, and social damage. It is not, in short, the benign substance that many users believe it to be. In a moment I'll discuss the results of those studies and how our attitudes about marijuana are changing.

First, though, a bit of history.

The Rise and Fall of Marijuana

Marijuana—*Cannabis sativa*—grows wild in the tropics. Its seeds are used as animal feed, its fiber for hemp rope, its oil for paint. Mostly, though, it's used to get high. As a weed, marijuana doesn't need a whole lot of cultivation. And unlike cocaine, you don't have to go through an elaborate chemical process to get a usable drug out of it. Just pick the leaves, light up, and that's it.

Use of marijuana dates back at least 2,000 years before the Christian era. Ancient Chinese, Indians, Middle Easterners, Greeks, and Romans knew about marijuana and used it in religious ceremonies or as a medical treatment. About 600 years ago an Arab historian blamed marijuana for causing the decline of Egyptian society.

The Spanish brought marijuana to the New World in 1545 to use in making rope. Hemp was grown in early American settlements, including Jamestown, as early as 1611. George Washington even cultivated the plants at Mount Vernon, carefully noting the fact in his diary.

Beginning in the 1840s, marijuana was touted as an herbal cure and was included in the official list of medicines until 1942. Before then, several major pharmaceutical firms sold products that contained cannabis. Smoking hashish became a fashionable pastime in the latter nineteenth century. Its use spread in the 1920s, the era of jazz clubs and Prohibition.

But in 1937 marijuana was effectively outlawed by the federal Marijuana Tax Act. Several states set harsh criminal penalties for use of the drug. In Georgia, selling marijuana to a minor could lead to life imprisonment or even death. By the 1960s, though, marijuana emerged as the symbol of the countercultural revolution.

Use of the drug continued to escalate every year—that is, until 1979. That's another part of the good news: Marijuana use has been declining, or at least stabilizing, for more than a decade now. More on that later.

The Effects of Marijuana

The good news about marijuana isn't that we've suddenly discovered a way to make pot safe and nontoxic. In fact, marijuana is not one drug but a hundred active and inactive drugs in one. The good news is that we know now what smoking dope can do to the body and the brain. Forewarned, as they say, is forearmed. (For more about the effects of marijuana, see Table, page 116.)

The "High" Although marijuana is usually smoked—rolled into cigarettes called joints or crumbled into pipes—it can be added to baked goods such as brownies and eaten. The principal active ingredient in marijuana, THC, doesn't dissolve in water, so it is almost never injected.

Many drugs work by attaching themselves to special receptors along the surfaces of cells in the body. Such receptors allow only molecules that have a specific shape to link up and trigger a response. Recently, genetic researchers have identified the specific receptor in the brain that is the target for marijuana's active ingredient. This discovery ranks as one of the most important findings in marijuana research and may ultimately lead to a better understanding of how the drug works and how to stop it from working at all. We may one day find a drug that fits that receptor without triggering the high or blocks it from working, which would be a tremendous step forward in the treatment of marijuana addiction.

The high kicks in within minutes of smoking; just how high one gets depends on the THC content. Usually the high lasts up to four hours. Secondary effects of marijuana—including damage to the body and changes in mental ability—last much longer.

Users describe the high as a light-headed feeling accompanied by greater sensual awareness. Colors seem more vivid; music more profound. Sometimes marijuana produces hallucinogenic sensations, such as distortions in time or space. Because emotions are intensified, many users experience paranoia and anxiety. Pot stimulates appetite, to which anyone who has ever had the "munchies" after smoking will attest. Marijuana also acts as a sedative, causing users to lose motor control or to "zone out" and fall asleep while sitting or driving.

Psychological Effects Pot affects short-term memory. Users might try to express a profound thought but will forget what

SIGNS AND SYMPTOMS OF MARIJUANA USE

Behavioral Signs
- Memory problems
- Chronic lying about whereabouts
- Sudden disappearance of money or valuables from home
- Suspicious robbery or breaking and entering while family is away
- Rapid mood changes
- Abusive behavior toward self or others
- Panic attacks
- Frequent outbursts
- Hostility with lack of insight or remorse for this behavior
- Increasing secretiveness

Social Signs
- Loss of driver's license
- Driving while impaired
- Auto accidents
- Frequent truancy
- Loss of part-time job or job problems
- Underachievement over past six to 12 months
- Definite deterioration of academic performance
- Dropout of rigorous sports or other activities

Circumstantial Evidence
- Smell of marijuana on clothes
- Drugs or drug paraphernalia in room, clothes, or automobile
- Whereabouts unknown for 36 or more hours
- Drug terminology in school notebooks or in school yearbook
- Change in friends
- Definitive change in peer-group preference to those peers who lack purpose, are unmotivated, and may be known to use marijuana
- Change in hygiene and attire

Medical Symptoms
- Chronic fatigue and lethargy
- Chronic nausea or vomiting
- Chronic dry irritating cough, chronic sore throat
- Headaches
- Chronic conjunctivitis (red eyes), otherwise unexplained
- Chronic bronchitis
- Impaired motor skill and coordination

you just said or what they were saying before they reach the end of their sentence. A "conversation" between smokers can be like having two radios tuned to different and distant stations —lots of static, no communication. Trying to teach someone who is high is a waste of time, since marijuana impairs the brain's capacity to process and store information. Studies show that marijuana's impact on memory continues up to six weeks after smoking stops.

Long-term use of marijuana at high doses can produce a brain disorder that causes psychosis and delirium. People with this syndrome become disoriented and confused and experience hallucinations.

A common problem of marijuana use is the *amotivational syndrome,* prevalent in adolescents but also seen in adults. The syndrome is marked by fatigue, loss of interest in any activity, low motivation, apathy, poor judgment, low attention span, impaired ability to communicate, and inability to plan ahead. Because these symptoms can lead to such problems as sinking grades or loss of friends, feelings of guilt or loneliness often emerge as a by-product. As we saw, Bryce experienced the full brunt of the amotivational syndrome.

Because the main activity for kids is school, the amotivational syndrome severly disrupts the learning process. Not only does pot wipe out short-term memory, it "erases" any new information that tries to get stored in the brain. It erodes self-discipline, causing further drops in learning. Drug abusers frequently get in trouble with the law.

Physical Effects The THC in marijuana smoke passes through the lungs and circulates in the bloodstream to the brain. In December 1990, researchers announced that they had found the receptor in the brain that locks onto THC. It then gets stored in fat cells (including cells in the brain, testicles, and ovaries) from which it is released slowly. Thus, even though a person stops smoking, the drug may still affect the body for days afterward. Because THC doesn't dissolve in water, like cocaine or alcohol, it is eliminated much more slowly than those drugs. In fact, people who smoke more than once a week or so may never rid their bodies of THC.

A common myth about marijuana is that it is less dangerous

than tobacco. Bull! A couple of joints do as much damage to the lungs as a whole pack of cigarettes. Pot smoke has up to ten times the amount of tar found in cigarette smoke. Because dopers hold the smoke in a long as they can, the lungs are exposed to perhaps four times as much carbon monoxide and other poisonous substances as they would get from tobacco. In fact, marijuana poses as much risk to users as alcohol and cigarettes *combined!*

Use of marijuana, especially long-term use, can lead to impaired hand-eye coordination. In one study, 94 percent of people who had smoked pot failed a standard roadside sobriety test, even an hour and a half after their last drug use. Sixty percent of them still failed the test two-and-a-half hours after smoking. Many people intoxicated on marijuana deny—or are actually unaware—that they are high. I think this makes them even more dangerous than drunk drivers, since the effects of alcohol are comparatively short-lived and the drinker usually knows perfectly well he is drunk. Without a roadside Breathalyzer test the true impact of marijuana on our highways cannot be determined. In the meantime, Designated Driver and Don't Drink and Drive programs should be expanded to include marijuana and other drugs.

Other problems of marijuana use include infertility, increased heart rate, panic attacks, and sensory distortions that contribute to anxiety, paranoia, and depression. Because marijuana affects motor ability, users are prone to falls, car accidents, and difficulty handling machinery. Heavy marijuana users who try to quit experience such complications as irritability, nausea, and sleeplessness. To avoid these symptoms, they just keep right on lighting up, and the cycle continues.

Many smokers report frequent sore throats or upper respiratory problems such as bronchitis. That users are susceptible to infections indicates the impact marijuana can have on the immune system—the body's defense against bacteria and viruses. Pot smokers who also use injectable drugs are at higher risk of contracting infections from needles. Long-term immune impairment also raises the risk of cancer. We have had actual experience with lung cancer that appeared to be directly related to chronic marijuana smoking.

Evidence clearly shows that marijuana, especially in high doses and for prolonged periods, has a direct impact on sexual functioning. Dope affects the levels of reproductive hormones in both sexes. In males, it reduces testosterone, the hormone responsible for transforming boys into men—bones, bodies, facial hair, genitals, and voice. It also leads to a lower sperm count—up to 70 percent lower in some patients. (I can remember a call from a medical colleague who had gone to a fertility clinic for help in having a child. My colleague wanted to know why the fertility clinic asked about his alcohol and marijuana use.) Oddly, though, in young girls it *increases* testosterone, disrupting ovulation and the menstrual cycle and causing skin problems.

We don't know whether these hormonal changes reduce fertility or whether they just decrease libido. Either way, the result is the same: a lower rate of pregnancy. It's also uncertain whether marijuana's impact on sexual function disappears when use of the drug stops, or whether it persists for the long term. Some men with low sperm counts due to marijuana use return to normal after a month of abstinence; in others, however, low sperm count persists.

Studies show that marijuana use affects a developing fetus. There is a well-established link between a mother's marijuana use and her baby's low birth weight. We even have evidence, both from animal research and reports on humans, that maternal use of marijuana can lead to birth defects. It pollutes the baby with hundreds of untested chemicals and may rob the fetus of oxygen, causing impaired growth, prematurity, and brain damage. While there is no official Fetal Marijuana Syndrome (remember, it took centuries before Fetal Alcohol Syndrome was recognized), I feel confident that there will be—that is, if enough pregnant women choose to experiment with their unborn children.

Marijuana—"risk free"? Sure—just like riding over Niagara Falls in a barrel.

Impact on Personality Marijuana users, especially adolescents, frequently show patterns of behavior and memory that indicate their intellectual performance is dropping. Studies show that marijuana affects thought patterns, reduces memory of even the simplest things, lowers concentration, and robs the user of the ability to handle complex tasks. (As one antidrug message put it, "Why do you think they call it 'dope'?") Patients report that their marijuana use has led to depression, sexual problems, and disturbances in their personalities. Often their social lives deteriorate because of pot—they alienate themselves from friends and family. Performance on the job suffers. For many addicts, marijuana is seldom their only problem. Many are compulsive users of alcohol, cocaine, or other drugs.

As we've seen, marijuana is associated with poor academic performance, low motivation, delinquent behavior, problems with authority, and low self-esteem. Interestingly, though, most individuals had these problems long before they smoked their first joint. Whether marijuana use actually makes these problems worse has yet to be proved conclusively. One thing is certain: It doesn't make them any better.

Psychiatric Impact Many chronic marijuana users exhibit symptoms that, to the untrained eye, look like some other form of psychiatric illness. For example, some people react to pot with severe anxiety and panic attacks. Others become very suspicious and negative. A person with schizophrenia might exhibit symptoms after smoking dope. If someone abuses several drugs, a kaleidoscope of abnormal behavior might emerge.

Some people use marijuana in the belief that it will help them sleep or relieve their depression. Wrong! Marijuana can *cause* insomnia and depression. But in their ignorance users smoke more and more pot to try to relieve these problems, until the compulsive, addictive pattern takes root.

Treating these symptoms, rather than the underlying problem—marijuana addiction—is futile. Using antianxiety drugs won't work if the anxiety has been triggered by marijuana. Sleeping pills won't relieve insomnia caused by marijuana use. For these and other reasons, I'm a strong believer in accurate drug testing, not just to identify which drugs have been abused but to help determine what kind of treatment is called for.

Is Marijuana Addicting?

Yes. Addiction means the compulsive use of a drug despite adverse consequences. By that criterion alone, most of the patients we wean from marijuana are addicted. They had continued smoking heavily when common sense or logic would suggest moderation, if not outright abstinence—in spite of lung infections or other medical problems, trouble with school or family, the threat of legal punishment, or loss of a job. All marijuana addicts deny their addiction, rationalizing it as merely a response to external events or pressures. Addiction to marijuana is both psychological and physiological.

Many smokers build up a tolerance, which means that more drug is needed to produce the same effect. However, tolerance can emerge whether a person is technically addicted or not. Clues that tolerance is present include mood changes, rapid heartbeat, low blood pressure, changes in body temperature, lower pressure in the eyeballs, changes in brain waves, and slower response times.

The stage after tolerance is dependence. People are said to be dependent when they can't quit using the drug under their own power or without suffering withdrawal symptoms. Some of those symptoms are anxiety, depression, disturbances of sleep and appetite, irritability, tremor, sweating, nausea, muscle convulsions, and restlessness. When a marijuana habit leads to preoccupation—when drug use becomes a priority and affects virtually every choice and activity—and frequent relapse, we are dealing with an addiction.

For many people, use of the drug itself causes addiction. Having so much of a toxic chemical floating around causes physical and psychological changes that compel the user to continue seeking the drug. Other people, however, are genetically vulnerable to marijuana addiction. Unfortunately, we can't identify those people until after they've started smoking. The new high-potency pot may be as addictive as cocaine or hashish.

Of course, marijuana is not automatically addicting. One toke will not turn someone into a monster or precipitate a psychiatric crisis. Millions of people have smoked large amounts of pot and lived to tell about it. But they are by no means living proof of—nor an endorsement for—pot's safety. They are no more an expert in marijuana than the heroin user is an expert in heroin. (Both are experts in denial.) Millions of people have smoked cigarettes and *not* suffered from cancer. We don't allow cigarette companies to use their endorsements, since we know that cigarette smoking does cause cancer. In my position as a treatment specialist, I have seen how marijuana can lead to addiction and ruin lives. The earlier and heavier the use, the greater the behavioral problems and the greater the risk of other illicit drug use.

We are successful at treating marijuana addiction because we understand that our patients suffer from a physiological disorder, not just some kind of personality disorder or moral failing. I can see, for example, that many users may begin smoking marijuana in response to some kind of stress. But a true marijuana addict really can't stop using the drug, even when all of those stressors have disappeared. Marijuana reinforces its own use. As Alcoholics Anonymous has taught us, a person born predisposed to marijuana addiction can no more resist the drug through "willpower" than someone dying of thirst in a desert can resist water.

The Gateway

Just about everyone who uses hard drugs started off with marijuana. One early NIDA study found that 98 percent of cocaine users had also used marijuana, but that *none* of the non-marijuana smokers had used cocaine. The more frequent the use of marijuana, the greater the likelihood that a person will move on to try coke (see Graph on page 123).

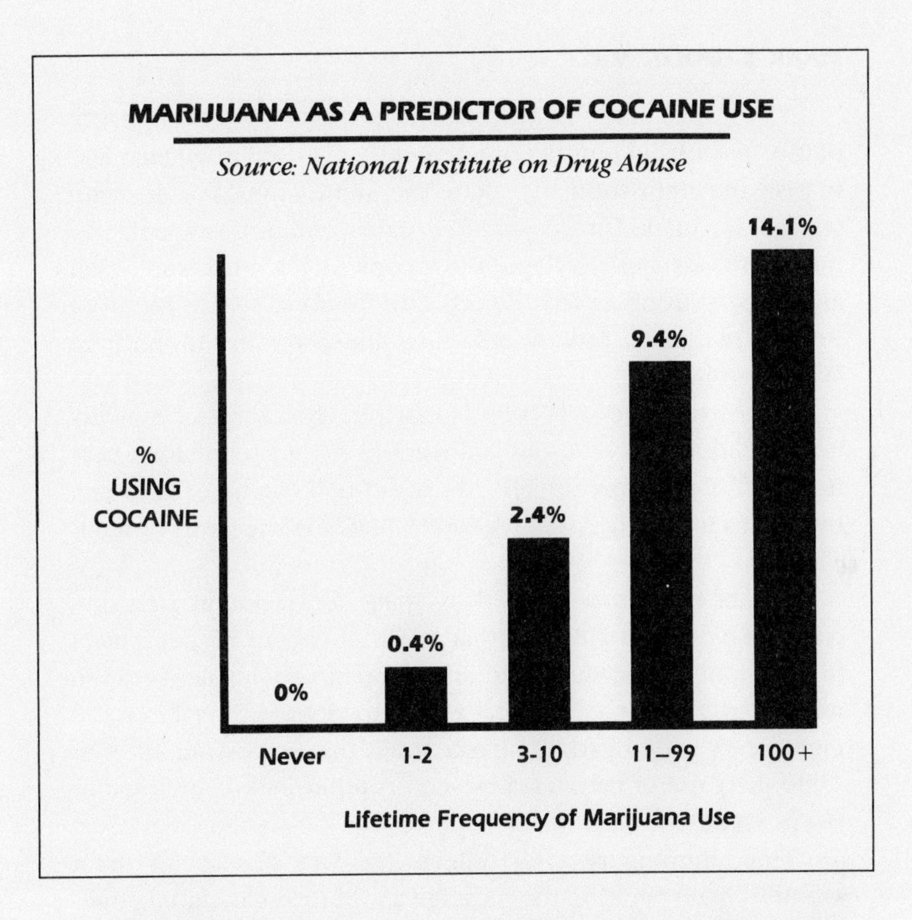

Coincidence? Or does marijuana use actually propel people into abusing other substances? There is growing evidence that marijuana does indeed cause the transition to other forms of addiction. For example, a survey by PRIDE showed that nearly half of high school seniors who use cocaine smoked marijuana by the age of 13 or under. As a rule, people who seek treatment for substance abuse don't identify marijuana as the source of their problem. In recent years, though, more and more patients are coming into treatment citing marijuana as their main drug of abuse.

The Good News About Marijuana: Changing Attitudes

In the 1960s, marijuana smoking became a badge of honor among those who challenged the traditional morals and values of the "Establishment." At one time to use or sell marijuana was to risk life imprisonment; since the sixties the laws of many states have made U-turns and decriminalized pot. Law enforcement officials basically ignored people who possessed small amounts. A group called NORML (the National Organization to Reform Marijuana Law) was formed and continues to lobby in Washington.

Meanwhile the THC content of pot increased as growers became more savvy about cultivation. A joint contained perhaps half of one percent THC during 1967's "Summer of Love"; by 1990 a joint might have 30 times that amount, or 15 percent THC.

Use of marijuana—fueled by these more potent strains—reached a peak in 1979. In that year only about 35 percent of high school seniors surveyed felt that people who smoke marijuana regularly were at "great risk." However, in 1987, a mere eight years later, nearly 75 percent felt that way. From 1978 to 1989 daily use of marijuana by seniors fell from 10.7 percent to 2.9 percent.

This stunning reversal reflects the fact that society as a whole is finally getting the message about drugs, including marijuana. Certainly the Partnership for a Drug-Free America and other media campaigns, the "Just Say No" program, and efforts of groups like PRIDE, the American Council for Drug Education, the 800-COCAINE helpline, the Scott Newman Foundation, Project DARE, and local school and community efforts have all contributed to this trend, not just in marijuana use but in use of all illicit drugs. It also shows just how powerful education about the risks of drug use can be.

Another positive trend is our increasing understanding of the biological nature of addiction. We have to be careful, though. Recently I tried to explain to the parents of a 16-year-old pot addict that her problem stemmed from a biochemical susceptibility, not from some lack of willpower. Somehow, though, they interpreted that to mean "There's nothing that can be done." I hastened to explain that, on the contrary, there's a *lot* we can do. The patient's will to get better is essential for treatment to succeed, but isn't enough in and of itself.

Psychiatrists have long been hampered by confusion about the exact nature of substance abuse disorders. Matters aren't helped any by the fact that the psychiatrist's "bible," the *Diagnostic and Statistical Manual, Third Edition-Revised* (DSM-III-R), lists criteria for diagnosing substance abuse that are essentially useless when it comes to spotting marijuana dependency.

DSM-III-R states that, in order to diagnose substance abuse, three rigid conditions must be met: a pattern of pathological use, impairment in social or occupational functioning, and a duration of at least a month.

Unfortunately, diagnosis is difficult with the addict's denial. Physicians must not stop at merely asking patients, their families, and their friends about drug use, but must also use drug testing when appropriate. If we sit around waiting for a patient, especially an adolescent, to admit to the DSM-III-R criteria before making our diagnosis, we are risking the patient's normal development—or even his life. The onset of marijuana dependence is often deceptive. We may not notice the pattern of use or the degree of impairment until it's too late. Another point: The DSM-III-R criteria are highly subjective. One doctor may decide that a slight drop in the patient's grades or frequent fights with family are enough to qualify as "social impairment," while another doctor may see these symptoms merely as typical "growing pains" and dismiss them.

Fortunately, more and more doctors—not just specialists and psychiatrists, but family doctors and general practice physicians—are becoming sensitized to their role in spotting and treating marijuana abuse. They now routinely include questions about drugs as a part of the diagnostic process, and may even order a urine drug screen. They rely on their own common sense and training, not on some rigid formula, to determine whether a drug problem exists. They don't just sit around waiting for a patient to deteriorate to a point beyond salvation. Instead they practice sound preventive medicine. They not only question the patient and the family about drug use, but they also use drug testing when appropriate.

In my speeches and writings, I do all I can to urge my

professional colleagues to be more aware of drug use. I would rather they err on the side of early diagnosis. At least that way they will be more likely to recognize earlier the presence of such warning signs as diminished school performance, impaired memory or concentration, or the amotivational syndrome. With an early diagnosis, treatment can be educational and lost time for normal adolescent development can be minimized. Urine testing would reveal whether patients had used marijuana within the previous weeks. Even when there is no blatant cause for suspicion, wider—even routine—use of such tests would help reveal evidence of drug use at an earlier and more easily treatable phase. Early identification could help prevent problems that might threaten the patient's health or the very stability of the patient's family. In addition, the early detection of drug use permits antidrug education to be used as a treatment resource. The sooner the diagnosis is made, the sooner treatment can begin and the greater the chance of success.

Not all the news is good, however. The trend toward decreased use of marijuana has apparently stabilized. A 1990 survey conducted by PRIDE indicates that marijuana and LSD may be increasing in affluent white neighborhoods. It appears that this increase may be tied to a surge of 1960s nostalgia. In addition, it's not increasing, but it's not getting much lower either. The age of first use of marijuana is dropping; and the younger the drug user, the greater the risk of lifelong physical or psychiatric reactions. That's why we should all campaign very hard for antidrug education programs beginning in kindergarten.

Also, much of the slowdown in marijuana use can be attributed to the wider availability and lower relative cost of cocaine and its derivative crack. Why pay up to $300 for the hard-to-get ounce of pot when for about a tenth that amount you can easily get ahold of a couple of rounds of crack? According to one Drug Enforcement Agency official, crack is now becoming the "gateway" drug of choice among a growing minority of addicts.

In the next chapter we'll take a detailed look at the nightmare that is cocaine.

CHAPTER SEVEN

Cocaine: The Clock Is Ticking

For the vast majority of Americans cocaine is dead. It isn't cool, it isn't sexy, it isn't funny. For most Americans, cocaine *is* passé, a thing of the past, something to be avoided at all costs. Unfortunately, not all of America shares in this good fortune. There are still places—especially in our urban areas—where cocaine continues to thrive and enslave entire communities. Nevertheless, on a grand scale, time is running out for cocaine.

I see cocaine fading into the past because the majority of Americans now share my view of cocaine, especially crack, as a deadly virus that ultimately kills its host. Even *Playboy*—once the self-proclaimed standard-bearer of the swinging sixties—described cocaine accurately: "(Cocaine) weakens us. It saps our productivity. It wastes our financial and spiritual resources. It makes us silly." A *Newsweek* reporter observed that there are now two Americas: "On one side, people of normal human appetites for food and sex and creature comforts; on the other, (cocaine users) who crave only the roar and crackle of their own neurons, whipped into a frenzy of synthetic euphoria."

Or, as one of my colleagues at Fair Oaks put it, coke makes sane people insane. When you talk to a person who's under the influence of cocaine, the conversation goes something like this: You say, "Now look, you're losing your health." And he says, "I've never felt better." You say, "You're losing your job." He says, "I'm still getting my paycheck, aren't I?" You: "You've lost all the respect of your coworkers." He: "You don't understand. I'm better than I ever was." The parasite that is cocaine saps a person's sense of perspective. Users lose all touch with reality.

Cocaine is truly an equal opportunity destroyer. Need proof? Look at the morning paper or the evening news. Rich or poor, educated or not, from the best of families or from no family at all—no one is immune. A former police chief admits to a 5-year-long cocaine addiction. A classical violinist is arrested for possession. High-level execs blow Fortune 500 fortunes on white powder. Crack-addicted parents beat infants to death. Whole neighborhoods become battlegrounds for drug lords' turf wars, and innocent bystanders die from the stray bullets. In Queens, drug dealers shot and killed a pregnant woman as their way of announcing that they had moved into a neighborhood and were open for business. Even Troy Donohue, TV star of the 1950s, sold his last piece of furniture to buy cocaine; homeless, he lived in New York's Central Park for a time.

The Good News About Cocaine

With all of this bad news is it possible to say anything good about cocaine?

Yes. For one thing, the sad fact that there are so many horror stories reported in the media has helped the message penetrate: *Coke is the thrill that kills.* At this point everyone in America has been directly affected by cocaine. No longer is the threat of drugs just some abstract problem that happens to "the other guy." The danger is real and immediate.

Consequently our attitudes are changing dramatically. In 1985, for example, only 34 percent of high school seniors surveyed agreed that cocaine could cause "great harm" if used just once or twice. By 1987, the figure was nearly 48 percent, and in the survey, the number of kids who knew that cocaine was "very harmful to health" was over 59 percent. From federal government programs to grass-roots movements in communities across the nation, people are transforming these new anti-drug attitudes into action to stop the spread of cocaine.

Here's proof: The number of people who used cocaine within the previous year fell from 12 million in 1985 to 6.2 million in 1988—a drop of 50 percent. In January 1988, over 40,000 people called the national helpline 800-COCAINE seeking help and information about drugs; in June 1990, this number dropped to 18,162. Today, over 91 percent of high school seniors disapprove of using cocaine once or twice.

More good news: We now know that cocaine addiction is a treatable disease. Recent breakthroughs in our understanding of how the drug attacks the brain have led to revolutionary new ways of counteracting its effects.

Thus there is much cause for hope: Education works. Prevention works. And treatment works.

The History of Cocaine

Cocaine comes from the leaves of coca plants—*Erythroxylon coca*—which thrive in the South American countries of Bolivia, Peru, and Colombia. The word coca derives from *kuka,* the Incan word for the plant.

Use of coca leaves may date as far back as 5,000 years before the Christian era. Archaeologists have also found evidence that, by around 1,500 BC, medicine men may have used a liquid coca-leaf compound as a topical anesthetic during a primitive form of brain surgery.

In the Incan empire (thirteenth to sixteenth century), coca was regarded as a sacred plant, a gift from the first Inca, the son of the Sun God. The leaves were used as good luck charms and as a part of initiation rites, weddings, and other religious ceremonies.

Then, as today in these regions, the coca leaf was chewed together with some kind of lime, which helps extract the stimulating ingredient, and a binding material. Chewing coca leaves is thought to strengthen the weak and help them forget their troubles.

When the explorer Amerigo Vespucci landed on an island off the coast of Venezuela in 1444 he noticed that the Indians' cheeks "bulged with the leaves of a certain green herb like cattle." After Pizarro conquered Peru in 1529, his government and the church tried to forbid the chewing of coca leaves, but without much success.

Apart from its religious use, coca leaves were thought to have many medicinal properties. The Indians seemed to use it the way we moderns use aspirin, coffee, tea, stimulants, and sedatives. Even today, coca is used by virtually all Peruvian peasants to ward off hunger, to protect against the cold, and as a remedy for stomach aches.

In the mid-1800s, scientists in Europe learned how to extract cocaine from the coca leaf. Soon afterwards people were using cocaine both for pleasure and as medicine. Angelo Mariani, a chemist from Corsica, bottled and sold an elixir he called Vin Mariani, a formula that included cocaine. Among those who endorsed the elixir were Thomas Edison and Pope Leo XIII.

In 1884, Sigmund Freud published a paper in which he declared that cocaine had many therapeutic uses, including the treatment of digestive disorders, cachexia (debility and malnutrition), and asthma. He also saw it as an aid in the treatment of morphine addiction, as an aphrodisiac, and as a local anesthetic. (He was right about cocaine in only one particular: It is an anesthetic.) Oh, yes: He did note in passing that excessive cocaine use could cause "physical and intellectual decadence," weakness, emaciation, and "moral depravity." But used in moderation, he concluded, cocaine was "more likely to promote health than impair it."

Freud is a classic example of how even a brilliant person who falls under the influence of cocaine can turn into a propagandist who is blind to its dangers.

A contemporary of Freud's, the Viennese physician Koller, pioneered the successful use of cocaine as an anesthetic in eye operations. Shortly afterwards, the Parke-Davis pharmaceuticals company declared that cocaine was potentially "the most important therapeutic discovery of the age" and began selling cocaine-containing products, such as coca cigarettes, used to treat throat infections. Cocaine was touted as a cure for everything from seasickness and tired blood to hemorrhoids and head colds.

In 1886, a patent-medicine maker from Atlanta created a drink made from coca leaves and kola nuts in a sweet, alcohol-free carbonated syrup, which he called "Coca-Cola" and which he promoted as a stimulant and a headache remedy.

Within an amazingly short time, though, evidence mounted that Freud's original conclusions were largely wrong. In 1887, Freud himself published a paper stating that cocaine was "a far more dangerous enemy to health than morphine." As the incidence of cocaine addiction rose—many doctors even became addicted themselves—its use became more and more restricted until finally it was seen as little more than a topical anesthetic. By the early 1900s the makers of Coca-Cola, aware of the public backlash, had removed the tiny dose of cocaine from their formulation.

In 1914, the United States mistakenly classified cocaine as a narcotic (it is a stimulant, not a depressant) and banned it, except for restricted medical applications. From the 1920s on it retained a certain notoriety among members of the upper class as "the champagne of pharmaceuticals"—high priced and chic. The tolerant attitudes toward illicit drugs in the 1960s, however, paved the way for the reemergence of cocaine that haunts us today.

I predict that one day the Smithsonian Institute will display the paraphernalia of the drug era. Seen as archaeological artifacts, these relics will reveal the changing patterns of drug use in recent years. In my imaginary display, I would have one area labeled "The Disco Era, circa 1975." At this time, when coke was relatively hard to get and expensive at $150 per gram, people thought it chic to wear gold-plated razor blades or cocaine spoons on chains around their necks. The dose of cocaine that such spoons held was laughably small. (For some of the cocaine addicts I have seen in my practice, use of a coke spoon to administer their daily intake would leave them no time to do anything else.) Soon spoons were replaced by lines—finely minced doses of cocaine about three inches long and served up on a mirror or glass tray. In another display case would appear needles and syringes, used to inject cocaine directly into the bloodstream.

This exhibit would also display another "innovation" in cocaine consumption: glass pipes for smoking cocaine. By the mid-1980s cocaine smoking had been prevalent for several years among users of the drug, but the process of extracting smokable cocaine—freebasing—was time consuming. It was also dangerous, as the comedian Richard Pryor discovered. He was badly burned when the ether he used to process cocaine exploded. Shortly afterwards drug users found they could extract cocaine base by a safe process using simple baking powder. The result is cocaine in the form of tiny colorless or cream-colored rocks. When burned in a pipe, these rocks make the crackling sound that gives crack its name.

Our hypothetical museum exhibit carries an important message: Within two decades what we consider a "dose" of cocaine has changed. Higher doses of more potent smoked cocaine, taken more frequently by younger and younger people, have transformed the experience of the drug, and its impact on society, tremendously.

Methods of Use

The way a person ingests coke determines its effects on the body. The Peruvian peasant who chews coca leaves or drinks coca tea is getting a relatively small dose. Even people who drank the truly classic Coke weren't at much risk. The amount of coke in Coke was pretty insignificant—much less than the dose taken from a cocaine spoon. Besides, it was an oral dose, and the oral route is about the least effective way to use cocaine. To my knowledge, there are no reported cases of people using Coca-Cola intravenously or lining up at the supermarket waiting for it to open so they could feed their Coke habit.

For years, of course, sniffing was the route of choice. But the nose acts as a natural barrier; less than half of the cocaine in a dose actually penetrates the nasal membrane. Because their high is diluted, and slower to begin, users feel compelled to try a different route and get more bang for their drug buck. Some users inject cocaine intravenously, but that method has obvious drawbacks. It's painful, it's hard to get syringes, and use of needles raises the risk of infectious disease, including AIDS, enormously.

Enter freebase. Freebase is smokable cocaine made by dissolving the white crystalline powder, cocaine hydrochloride, in a strong base. Smoking coke gives a quicker, more intense high than inhaling cocaine powder because the drug passes quickly and unhindered from the lungs to the bloodstream. Richard Pryor told audiences that the freebase high was instantaneous. He even noticed a kind of conditioned response: As soon as the pipe touched his mouth, he felt profoundly euphoric. In 1983, only 21 percent of callers to 800-COCAINE said they were freebasing; by 1987, that number jumped to 56 percent.

Crack is simply freebase that's been mass-produced. Crack melts at 98 degrees Centigrade—much lower than the melting point of cocaine powder—and turns into smoke at any temperature higher than that. Crack produces an intense high in eight seconds or less. The high lasts only between 5 and 15 minutes, during which the user feels more confident, more intelligent, more in control, and sexier.

But the abrupt high is followed by an abrupt crash. Both to repeat the high and to avoid that crash, users are driven to take another dose immediately. And another. And off they go down the road to tolerance, dependence, and ultimately, addiction. Calls to 800-COCAINE show that, while the typical coke snorter used the drug for up to five years before becoming addicted, a crack user can be hooked within two to six months —or even sooner. In contrast, a person might use alcohol for ten years before becoming addicted.

Some users, not willing to let bad enough alone, combine cocaine with other drugs. Those savvy cocaine lords south of the border have created a new market for their drug by packaging crude cocaine with marijuana or tobacco in a highly addictive drug called *bazuco*—bazooka, as we know it here. Some users mix coke with heroin to control the postcoke crash. This combination, known as the speedball, killed John Belushi. As crack spreads, so does the use of the speedball. Close to 90 percent of cocaine users also use some other form of drug, including tobacco, alcohol, and marijuana. Many crack users, both occasional smokers and long-term addicts, turn to these drugs, or even heroin, to extend the high and cushion the crash.

Cocaine Use Today

In 1976, only about 20 tons of cocaine made its way into this country. By 1990, up to 80 tons, worth more than $55 billion, was imported a year. Seldom sold in 100 percent pure form, adulterated coke sells for anywhere from $40 to $140 a gram—as much as ten times the price of gold.

The increasing availability has changed the demographic patterns of cocaine use. As I mentioned, for most of this century use was largely limited to affluent people who could afford to pay for the drug. A few users could be found among the poor and other groups, such as artists and musicians. In a survey conducted in 1983 among callers to the 800-COCAINE helpline, we found that half of the callers had at least some college education, and that 52 percent were earning more than $25,000 a year.

Such findings confirmed the image of cocaine as the drug of choice among the elite, the "yuppies," the people in high-profile, high-power careers. As a "success drug," cocaine seduces intelligent, competent people because it magnifies the qualities we associate with achievement. Coke users report having more energy, less need for sleep, enhanced self-esteem, and high ambition—practically a prescription for such people as executives, money traders, entertainers, and doctors, who need to feel in control and on top of the world.

Before 1985, less than half of the callers reported using cocaine daily—most took it only once or twice a week. Importantly, though, even at this relatively low intake, 63 percent of those calling considered themselves addicted. Over 70 percent stated that they preferred cocaine to food, and half would rather use the drug than have sex. One out of ten reported that they had attempted suicide.

The picture started to change with the arrival of crack. Surveys conducted between 1985 and 1987 showed that the typical cocaine user was now uneducated; 80 percent earned less than $25,000. It was clear that crack, priced as low as $3 to $5 a dose, had spread into poor urban regions and was even being used by school kids who previously couldn't afford drugs.

By 1989, crack's effect had become even more pronounced. Now, less than 50 percent of those who called were employed. (See Table on page 136.)

Recent surveys have also highlighted the fallacy of so-called recreational cocaine users. A June 1990 survey of callers to 800-COCAINE found that even callers using cocaine once or twice a week (i.e., the "recreational" users) report severe problems stemming from their drug use. In fact, there is little difference between the "recreational user" and the "everyday addict":

- Sixty-seven percent of the "recreational users" have incomes under $25,000, compared to 57 percent of the "everyday addicts."
- Fifteen percent of the "recreational users" and 19 percent of the "everyday addicts" are married.
- Eight percent of the "recreational users" are college graduates, compared to 14 percent of the "everyday addicts."

The only major area where the two groups differ is in length of cocaine use. Forty-one percent of the "everyday addicts" have been using drugs for more than five years, compared

COMPARISON OF 800-COCAINE SURVEYS 1983–1989

	1983	1985	1987	1989
College Education	50%	50%	16%	30%
Freebase/Crack	21%	30%	56%	55%
Intranasal Use	61%	52%	24%	39%
Unemployment	16%	16%	54%	55%
Income 25k/yr & up	52%	27%	20%	34%
Average Age	31	28.5	27	28
Males	67%	58%	63%	65%
Females	33%	42%	37%	35%

to only 25 percent of the "recreational users." Without an educational or treatment intervention, and given enough time these "recreational users" will almost certainly turn into everyday addicts.

Crack has upped the ante in cocaine addiction. The levels of use are higher, the plunge into addiction faster than ever before. One patient told me that within six months he had gone from being a successful businessman to someone who grovelled on his hands and knees in crack houses in rotten neighborhoods to pick up crumbs of crack others had left behind. Another said she couldn't be bothered dropping her daughter off at school. Instead she took her daughter along on her drug forays to her friend's apartment. "The kid would sit crying while I crawled into my pipe and disappeared," she recounted. Officials at daycare centers, after-school programs, and hospitals in urban neighborhoods state that up to 70 percent of the children they see are being raised by older relatives, typically grandmothers, as their crack-addicted parents abandon them in their search for euphoria.

Effects of Cocaine

Euphoria Of course, people use cocaine to get high. That feeling of euphoria comes from a burst of cocaine to the brain. You don't get it just from having high levels of cocaine circulating in the blood.

The sense of euphoria is related to the primitive feeling known as "fight or flight." Cocaine stimulates the secretion of adrenaline (epinephrine), a hormone that stimulates the central nervous system and makes people feel alert, full of self-confidence, and invincible. That's fine if you're a jungle primate being threatened by an approaching tiger. But without that very real threat, your body is all charged up with no place to go.

The euphoria is so intense—some IV users even report experiencing orgasm—that vivid memories of the experience get burned into the brain. Whenever users feel down, these memories get stirred up and haunt them until they seek out, and use, more coke. The act of using cocaine is so highly rewarded by the body that the drug reinforces its own use. In other words, the euphoria induced by cocaine causes a person to shift immediately to using high doses in binges. Animals allowed to self-administer cocaine will do so until they die.

Another reinforcing factor: Some coke users initially become more energetic and productive, a change that draws positive comments from other people. As Patricia, a 33-year-old ad copywriter told me, "After I started using coke, my boss said she was impressed with my performance and would put me in for a raise and a promotion. I knew I had to keep snorting, or I'd never be able to live up to her expectations." Such social reinforcement can sometimes trigger the slide into addiction.

We see the same thing in many athletes, entertainers, and public figures who become cocaine addicts. They work hard to earn the adulation of a crowd and attain a sense of well-being and control—what we call the "performance high." That feeling can come from a touchdown in the Super Bowl or winning an election. But the feeling is so exhilarating that these people want to experience it again and again. That urge has become known as "chasing the high"—in other words, addiction.

The pleasure centers in the brain aren't just there to make life fun, although they help do that. Pleasure is a biologically programmed response that tells the body something good is happening, something that will enhance survival. Sex is good because it preserves the species, eating likewise. But coke tricks the body into thinking that some basic survival drive is being gratified. But the body's pleasure centers can only take so much stimulation. In time, cocaine wears down the pleasure centers, which explains why stimulants eventually lose their potency. Euphoria is replaced by anxiety, paranoia, and depression. Heavy users describe the experience as being an emotional roller coaster ride and notice that they have become unable to enjoy anything—food, entertainment, even sex.

As my Fair Oaks colleague Irl Extein observes, using cocaine is like driving with your foot full on the accelerator. You give the car a lot of gas and race around at dangerously high speeds for a while. Soon, though, you run out of gas. No matter how furiously you pump the pedal or grind the starter, the car slows down. You've reached that stage of coke use marked by chronic depression.

After the high, the nervous system relaxes, but the cocaine remains in the bloodstream. Eventually toxic effects build up. Common side effects include decreased sleep, loss of appetite, hyperactivity, aggressiveness, feelings of grandeur, poor social judgment, and malnutrition.

A list of the signs and symptoms of cocaine use appears in the Table on page 139. Often, the less clinical symptoms of cocaine use are the most revealing. Clues like changes in friends, loss of interest in activities, poor grades, changes in dress, mood, or other subtle behavioral shifts should set off an alarm. The earlier such signs are spotted, the better the chance that treatment will be effective.

Cocaine Addiction Up until around 1985, the "experts" still weren't sure whether cocaine was an addicting drug. It took the devastating impact of crack to convince some people of the awful truth. Cocaine is so addicting that many dealers won't even use it because they know that all of their profits would literally go up in smoke if they did.

As I mentioned in Chapter Four, addiction to cocaine, or any drug, usually takes place in discrete stages: experimentation, social-recreational use, preoccupation, and dependency. Some experts use a dollar figure to help recognize addiction in a patient; Dr. Extein, for example, defines a moderate addiction

SIGNS & SYMPTOMS OF COCAINE USE

PHYSICAL AND MENTAL

- Increased or decreased tolerance for alcohol or drugs
- Red face, red nose
- Bumps and bruises from falling, etc.
- Puffiness of face or extremities
- Sudden vision difficulties
- Swollen nasal membrane
- Chest and heart problems including bronchitis, changed heart rhythms, heart failure
- Enlarged liver
- Frequent infections
- Digestive problems
- Lingering colds and flu
- High blood pressure
- Signs of bad nutrition
- Tremors
- Blackouts
- Changes in reflexes
- Loss of coordination
- Dizziness
- Confusion and slow comprehension
- Slurred speech
- Memory loss
- Anxiety or depression
- Delirium
- Hallucinations
- Insomnia
- Impotence
- Craving for sweets or a complete avoidance
- Loss of appetite

BEHAVIOR AND SOCIAL

- Increased reliance on drugs
- Family problems
- Financial difficulties
- Frequent change of jobs, lateness, other job-related problems
- Car accidents
- Increased legal problems from behavior
- Suicidal behavior
- Violent behavior
- Suspiciousness
- Unusually passive behavior
- Increased severity of usual neurotic symptoms

as a habit that costs up to $50 a day, and a severe addiction as one costing between $50 and $200 a day or more.

Addiction to the drug is expressed as a craving—a kind of "hunger." Actually, we now know there are three stages of cocaine cravings.

Immediate craving appears as soon as the high wears off. Users feel irritable, depressed, and agitated, and want nothing more than to feel good again. Thus they use up their entire supply of drugs in a futile effort to avoid the unavoidable crash. As one former user noted, "People are discovering that the principal thing one does with cocaine is run out of it." This phase, marked by fatigue, depression, increased appetite, and oversleeping, can last up to four days.

Intermediate craving begins when the worst of the crash is over. It persists for up to ten weeks, but usually lessens over time. If they can ride it out, most users will learn to overcome their craving. It takes a lot of willpower to do so, however, and most people can't make it through the weeks of this phase without relapsing. As we'll see in Chapter 13, part of effective treatment for cocaine addiction involves strategies to block cravings during this crucial time.

The last type is the *provoked craving,* triggered by anything from the sight of talcum powder to a crack pipe or a mirror. One recovering patient, accustomed to driving into New York to score crack, reported that he relapsed one night after driving through the Holland Tunnel. For this reason, treatment needs to address the patient's entire life-style and environment. It does no good to treat people and return them to homes where parents, spouses, or siblings continue to use drugs. The temptations are everywhere, and they're just too great.

In fact, no obvious temptation (like talcum powder) may be necessary to trigger the urge to use cocaine. Relapse may even be linked to subtle changes in the brain. For example, Bob Post at the National Institute of Mental Health found that cocaine can cause a *kindling* response in the brain. Apparently this kindling response occurs after parts of the brain are repeatedly stimulated by cocaine. Repeat stimulation lowers the brain's activity threshold—levels of stimulation that had previously been tolerated will now trigger a reaction. If stimulation from cocaine is repeated enough times, changes in the brain may actually occur spontaneously with no cocaine consumption being necessary (a picture of cocaine or even something that smells like cocaine could be the trigger.) This is the kindling response that may lead to the urge to use cocaine and lead to relapse.

Different people experience different degrees of susceptibility to cocaine. True, some people who use coke never become addicted. But we know that adolescents are particularly susceptible. Adults average four years of coke snorting before their function deteriorates and addiction takes over; in teenagers, the time lag averages just a year and a half. But using coke in the hopes that you'll be one of the lucky few who won't become addicted is like playing Russian roulette using a six-shooter with five bullets. I know of some cases of people who have used stimulants in high doses for long periods and who still notice the effects—low energy, inability to feel pleasure, and persistent cravings—for as long as *ten years* after their last binge.

The Nuts and Bolts of Addiction

Innovative research at Fair Oaks and at other centers has led to the important discovery that cocaine produces addiction by interfering with three vital chemicals found in the brain. These chemicals, the neurotransmitters, are norepinephrine, dopamine, and epinephrine.

Neurotransmitters relay information across the gaps between nerve cells. As stimulants, they control our perception of, and our response to, emotions and feelings of pain and pleasure. Normally the cells in the brain retain adequate stores of these neurotransmitters and release them when needed.

We now know that cocaine acts by screwing up the natural regulatory system and tricking the brain into releasing its supplies of neurotransmitters. Once released, these chemicals—particularly dopamine—cause nerve cells to fire, creating the rush of euphoria that the user is seeking. The problem is that cocaine doesn't bother to tell the cells to *stop* releasing dopamine. Eventually the cells deplete their entire supply. Another problem is that usually the cells reabsorb the dopamine once it has done its job of activating the nerves. But coke interferes with this recycling. Thus cocaine puts a double-whammy on the brain: It triggers the release of its supply of neutrotransmitters, and prevents it from reusing that supply. I call this model of addiction the dopamine depletion hypothesis. Mike Kuhar at the National Institute has even identified what he believes is the cocaine receptor on the Dopamine neurons in the brain.

Their supply of neurotransmitters gone, users must take more and more cocaine to achieve the same rush they got with a previous dose. Their tolerance leads to increased use, which triggers the descent into addiction. But when they try to stop, they discover just how powerful, and necessary, the need for a functioning neurotransmitter system is. At this point the brain doesn't even have a big enough supply of chemicals to get it through a normal day. And without neurotransmitters, the brain experiences withdrawal—the intense feelings of depression and physical pain associated with craving. Thus cocaine addicts find they now need their drug not to feel high but to keep from feeling bad—to fend off the horrors of coke cravings.

This process of addiction takes place regardless of whether the coke is snorted, smoked, or shot into the veins. As I've said, however, the effects of smoking or injecting coke are so intense, and occur with such rapidity, that the length of time before the user becomes addicted is shortened dramatically.

The good news about the discovery of dopamine depletion is that it has led to an innovative new way of initially treating cocaine addiction with bromocriptine, a medication that temporarily replaces the body's need for dopamine. Use of this drug masks or totally eliminates early cocaine withdrawal symptoms, and is the first pharmacological tool we used to help users tolerate total abstinence after years of using cocaine. By lessening cocaine's early withdrawal symptoms, bromocriptine helps decrease dropout rates in treatment. (See Box on pages 144–45.)

Medical Complications of Cocaine Use

Cocaine makes you blind. I don't necessarily mean it robs you of your vision, although there is some risk of that. I mean that users refuse to see the threat to their health that cocaine poses. The myth holds that cocaine is a "safe" drug. The truth is quite different: The side effects of cocaine are very serious, and often deadly.

To some extent, the effects of cocaine depend on the route of administration. Snorting is less intense and effective than smoking; cocaine injected intravenously is the most potent of all. Contrary to myth, users can overdose by any route, including snorting.

As with crack, the high from IV use is short lived. Thus users who prefer this route must shoot up frequently, increasing their risk of hepatitis, bloodstream infections, and bacterial endocarditis (inflammation of the lining of the heart). Even though the rate of IV use has dropped to about 9 percent, the incidence of AIDS among 800-COCAINE callers rose from 1 percent to 4 percent between 1987 and 1989. Some complications of IV use are due to infected needles or "mistakes" made during injection, while other complications come from shooting powerful and possibly tainted drugs directly into the blood.

Some medical complications arise from the fact that cocaine is often "cut" with substances ranging from quinine and lactose (milk sugar) to talc and cornstarch. And despite the myth, crack is not pure cocaine. If the original cocaine powder contains impurities, so will its crack derivative, and in even higher concentrations. Neither the cutting agents nor the water the drug is mixed with for injection is sterile. Putting this stuff into the body risks having it block a blood vessel or poison the tissues where it accumulates. It may also send a smorgasbord of bacteria, fungi, and viruses into circulation.

Peering Into the Cocaine Brain

Until recently, researchers were limited in their ability to understand cocaine's effects upon the human brain. After all, the skull posed a rather formidable obstacle. However, a wide variety of high-tech diagnostic imaging techniques have allowed scientists to safely look inside the brain of cocaine users without disturbing a hair. These techniques include:

Computerized Axial Tomography (CT Scan): The CT scan works by measuring low levels of radiation after it passes through tissue. Radioactive rays are affected by the density of tissue; the CT scan first uses external detectors to measure these altered levels and then uses a computer to reconstruct images based upon the results.

CT scans of subjects with a history of multiple drug abuse have revealed structural brain damage. This brain damage most likely stems from the hemorrhages and blood clots that have been associated with the abuse of drugs. There has even been one report of a newborn baby developing a blood clot in the brain within 24 hours of birth. The baby's mother had taken 1 gram of cocaine 15 hours before delivery!

Positron Emission Tomography (PET): PET is a recently developed technique that provides high-resolution, three-dimensional images of the brain. Radioactive compounds—selected for their ability to concentrate in different areas in the brain—are intravenously injected. Areas in the brain where these compounds collect can then be mapped by detectors. Compounds have been developed for their ability to measure a wide range of activities, including oxygen metabolism, cerebral blood flow, and neurotransmitter levels.

PET studies that measure the cerebral blood flow of chronic cocaine users have found areas in the brain where blood flow is severely restricted. These findings support the theory that drug abuse leads to strokes and blood clots in the brain.

Other studies using PET techniques have reported that cocaine decreases the brain's metabolism of glucose, a condition that occurs in severely depressed patients. This decreased glucose metabolism may partially explain the depression that accompanies a "cocaine crash."

continued

Perhaps most significantly, cocaine's effect on neurotransmitters—specifically the dopamine depletion hypothesis I described on page 144—has been documented by PET. Studies have shown that chronic cocaine administration can lead to long lasting and severe physical changes in the brain. Recent studies show that prolonged dopamine depletion may last up to two months or longer.

While PET Scan techniques are undoubtedly useful in psychiatry, they may never achieve the subtlety and incredible sophistication necessary to uncover the minute details of the brain or find its "euphoric center."

Complications also depend on the dose of the drug. Different people experience different susceptibility to cocaine. Some people are born lacking the enzyme (the name, for the record, is pseudocholinesterase) whose main function is to seek out and destroy toxins such as cocaine. For such people, even the small amounts of cocaine used for anesthesia during surgery can be fatal.

Let's take a quick tour of the body. At each stop we'll see how cocaine can do its dirty work.

Nasal passages: Cocaine constricts the blood vessels. Snorting can thus cause the vessels in the nose to wither and die, leading to rhinitis—inflammation of the nasal membrane and chronic nasal discharge. (Rhinitis is why so many chronic coke users go around sniffling all the time.) Over time coke can destroy the septum and lead to nasal deformity that requires plastic surgery. Deep-tooting with a tube can cause inflammation of the sinuses.

Lungs: You name it, coke'll do it to you. One in four callers to 800-COCAINE reports suffering from respiratory problems —anything from chronic cough and bronchitis (an inflammation of the main airways) to inflammation of the trachea, hoarseness, loss of voice, and wheezing. Many coke smokers cough up blood or a tar-like residue.

The impact of cocaine on the lungs' ability to function is as disastrous as if the user had inhaled gasoline. The problem is worsened because crack smokers inhale as deeply as they can, and hold the smoke in for as long as possible, to get the biggest high. Once weakened, the lungs lose their ability to remove poisonous gases from the body. The presence of smoke, or the smoker's frequent and violent coughs, ruptures tiny air spaces in the lung, allowing air to leak into lung tissue, leading to severe chest pain. Because cocaine constricts small blood vessels, it interferes with the flow of oxygen into the blood, leading to shortness of breath, rapid or irregular breathing, gasping, and accumulation of fluid in the lungs. Many of these changes, including loss of lung elasticity and bronchitis, can be permanent. I find it strange that people who wouldn't dream of smoking cigarettes won't hesitate to smoke crack.

Recently a new syndrome became part of medical terminology: crack lung. People with this condition have the same symptoms seen in pneumonia—severe chest pains, breathing problems, and high temperatures. Of course, crack lung is caused not by a virus or bacteria but by inhaling a poisonous substance. Thus patients show up in the emergency room with what looks like pneumonia, but which doesn't appear on X rays and which won't respond to any of the standard treatments. (Anti-inflammatory drugs, however, do help relieve symptoms of crack lung.) People with crack lung can suffer oxygen starvation or loss of blood—and die.

Anyone showing symptoms of crack lung, or the cardiac symptoms I'll describe next, must go quickly to the nearest emergency room.

Heart: Cocaine use has been linked to virtually every type of heart disease, including arrhythmias, heart attacks, coronary atherosclerosism, and congestive heart failure.

Cocaine users almost universely report an increase in heart rate minutes after using the drug. This increase in heart rate, called tachycardia by physicians, is classified as an arrhythmia. Arrhythmias are irregular heartbeats that can lead to serious, even fatal, medical complications. For example, irregular heartbeats can lead to a condition called fibrillation, where the heart muscles beat uncontrollably. Left untreated, fibrillation is almost always fatal. Obviously, not every cocaine user dies from an irregular heartbeat. But anyone who subjects his heart to the power of cocaine is playing Russian roulette with his life.

Cocaine's effect upon the heart doesn't stop with an irregular heartbeat. Research suggests that cocaine can induce spasms in the heart muscle that can cause a heart attack, even in otherwise healthy individuals. Cocaine can cause angina pain and should not be mixed with strenuous exercise.

Cocaine can cause heart attacks in other ways. For example, cocaine increases oxygen demand in the heart muscles while simultaneously restricting blood flow (and decreasing the body's ability to deliver oxygen). Consequently, cocaine users may develop a condition called *silent myocardial ischemia* that may lead to valuable heart muscle cells dying from lack of oxygen. In essence, cocaine speeds the heart while making it difficult for the heart to supply itself with oxygen. Mix this state with a little exercise or competitive sport and *whammo!*

Cocaine also has the unfortunate side effect of accelerating *coronary atherosclerosis* in patients with premature artery disease. Atherosclerosis is the plaque that builds up on the inside walls of an artery, thereby narrowing the artery. The narrowed arteries further reduce blood flow and increase the likelihood of a blood clot that blocks blood flow (and causes a heart attack). Cocaine may also affect platelets, the disk-shaped structures in the blood responsible for coagulation. According to this theory, cocaine causes platelets to form blood clots.

Because cocaine-induced heart irregularities are so common among the young, I always urge physicians to consider cocaine abuse in the diagnosis of otherwise healthy patients.

In addition, cocaine elevates blood pressure, sometimes to the point where spontaneous bleeding occurs in patients with otherwise normal blood pressure. This elevated blood pressure strains the heart, and may even underline many incidents of large stroke or small leaks of blood in the brain, associated with cocaine use.

Endocrine System: Cocaine intoxication can cause the thyroid to overproduce hormones. These in turn can produce the syndrome of high blood pressure, sweating, rapid heartbeat, tremor, anxiety, and high body temperature seen in hyperthyroidism. Conversely, the cocaine "crash" results in the symptoms of hypothyroidism: low energy, depression, weight gain, excessive sleepiness, and a slowing down of activity, including speech.

Other Effects: After cocaine's initial aphrodisiac effects have worn off, many patients report having less, or no, interest in sex. Those who are still interested find they can't perform nearly as well.

Studies find that cocaine significantly reduces not just total sleep, but the amount of time spent in REM sleep—the dreaming phase. Many addicts report that their sleep is disturbed by cocaine-related dreams, especially when they are going through withdrawal. It's not enough that their every waking hour is focused on the drug; their sleep is haunted by it as well.

Many users neglect their hygiene; surprisingly, dental problems are the most often reported medical complication among patients at Fair Oaks.

Frighteningly, perhaps one out of eight callers to 800-COCAINE report having had an epileptic-like seizure due to cocaine use.

Death: Death from cocaine can happen to anyone from a first-time user to a seasoned veteran of drug abuse, regardless of dose or route of administration.

Cocaine causes death in several ways: medical emergencies, such as those I've described above; accidental death, caused by anything from driving while zonked to getting shot during a drug deal (or being shot as an innocent passerby—or, in the horrid slanguage of the street, a "mushroom"); homicide; and suicide. Brain deaths from seizure or respiratory failure are usually associated with high doses; cardiac deaths can often occur even at seemingly low doses. Officially, a fatal dose of cocaine in humans is put at 1.2 grams, but there are reports of people who died after a dose of 20 milligrams—one sixtieth of the supposedly fatal dose. At first, signs that death is on its way include excitement, anxiety, restlessness, and confusion. Often the person faints and convulses. Death is usually rapid, a mixture of central nervous system stimulation, respiratory depression, and cardiovascular collapse.

Since 1982–1983, as cocaine use has risen, the number of cocaine-related emergency room visits has jumped 500 percent. We've also seen a corresponding rise in fatal reactions to cocaine. The good news is, we now recognize that cocaine causes severe medical complications. The bad news is, there's damn little we can do for patients who are in such danger that they have to be brought to the ER.

Psychiatric Effects

In describing the medical complications of cocaine, I feel like a pitchman on one of those late night TV ads: "Yes, with cocaine, you get heart problems, lung problems, and death. But wait! You get a basketful of mental and emotional problems as well! Depression! Anxiety! Paranoia! And many, many more!"

In a recent 800-COCAINE survey, 35 percent of callers reported experiencing chronic depression. Depression is, in fact, the most common long-term problem we see in our patients who abuse cocaine. Cocaine users can become so profoundly depressed that they commit suicide. Cocaine also causes anxiety. Often the anxiety becomes so severe that users turn to depressant drugs, such as alcohol, for relief. Many coke users experience tactile or visual hallucinations. One common hallucination is the feeling that live insects are crawling on the skin, an experience so widespread that it's even earned a name: the "coke bugs." Paranoia, especially fear of the police, is also rampant. Even people who have never had a psychiatric problem experience hyperactivity, irritability, severe panic, and even an overwhelming fear of impending death as their coke binge continues.

There's no doubt that cocaine can cause psychiatric problems. But it's also true that many people who originally suffer from these problems turn to drugs, including cocaine, as a form of self-treatment. For example, cocaine users in one study said that they were plagued with chronic self-doubt, apprehension, low energy, and insomnia occurring in the early part of the sleep cycle. These people were drawn to cocaine because it energized them and helped them overcome their low energy, do better at work, and relate better to other people.

Evidence is mounting that people who experience certain emotional patterns choose cocaine, whereas people who have a different pattern will tend to abuse other drugs. At Fair Oaks we found that 20 percent of patients who chronically abused cocaine also met the criteria for bipolar disorder (including manic depression and its less severe version known as cyclothymic disorder), but that only one percent of patients who abused opiates met these criteria. Such findings suggest that people with these disorders are predisposed to choose cocaine as their substance of abuse. Even after they have been detoxified, up to half of the cocaine addicts we treat meet the criteria for major depressive disorder, suggesting that the problem existed before they became substance abusers. In contrast, only ten percent or less of detoxified alcoholics meet these criteria.

One in ten callers to 800-COCAINE reports feeling paranoia. One Fair Oaks patient told us that whenever she tooted up, she began to believe there were people hiding in her oven and digging a secret tunnel under her apartment. Whenever she turned to her stereo, she heard people laughing and saying, "We've got you now!"

Some people who suffer from hyperactivity, restlessness, or an attention-deficit disorder report that cocaine helps calm them down and improves concentration and performance. This is odd, since cocaine is a stimulant and should, by rights, produce the opposite effect. Part of the good news, as we'll see in subsequent chapters, is that patients with cyclical mood disorders and attention-deficit disorders often quit using cocaine and other drugs when treated with the right medications.

Violence

In addition to its physical and mental effects, crack has what I call "social side effects." Among the more frightening of these is its incredible ability to stir up violence in its users. Crack smokers become irritable, suspicious, and extremely negative. They develop a very short fuse, and will lash out at another person at the slightest provocation. Some of that violence is linked to the dangerous and highly competitive business of drug dealing itself, including fear of the police. Some is related to the drug's pharmacologic effects, and some is just plain random, unfocused aggression.

In past years, the violence associated with drug use was a result of the agonies of withdrawal or a part of crimes committed to support one's habit. But today, callers to 800-COCAINE report that they become violent *while high or coming down from the drug.* Nearly half of the cocaine users responding to one of our surveys admitted that they committed violent crimes or aggressive acts, and two-thirds of those said they did so while using, as compared to when they were abstinent. Of those violent acts, 25 percent were violent arguments; 20 percent physical fights; 13 percent robberies; 7 percent domestic violence. Other crimes included child abuse, rape, even murder. One out of six told us that his cocaine habit had led him to carry a gun. Over 80 percent of crack users believed that crack caused their violent behavior.

Here's something guaranteed to keep you awake at night: In the first three months of 1989, 76 percent of all people arrested in New York City had traces of cocaine in their urine. (In contrast, only 13 percent had traces of marijuana.) Keep in mind that cocaine is usually eliminated from the body within days but that marijuana can be detected weeks after its last use. The fact that so many people arrested revealed traces of cocaine indicates that they had used it very recently and shows a striking link between use of the drug and their crime (see table on page 152 for drug-use rates of arrestees in our major cities.)

RATES OF DRUG-USE ARRESTS IN MAJOR CITIES

City	% Positive Any Drug	2+ Drugs	Cocaine	Marijuana	Amphetamines	Opiates	PCP
MALES							
San Diego	85	48	42	44	35	18	6
New York	80	30	76	13	—	17	3
Philadelphia	79	33	74	24	—	10	3
Wash., D.C.	72	36	65	13	0	14	22
Detroit	68	17	54	24	0	7	0
Dallas	67	29	50	34	4	7	2
New Orleans	66	29	59	26	0	6	6
Cleveland	66	22	56	22	0	4	3
St. Louis	64	26	47	24	1	4	9
Kansas City	60	15	44	22	2	2	2
Portland	54	21	36	27	7	9	0
San Antonio	51	23	24	28	6	14	0
Indianapolis	50	14	26	30	0	2	—
FEMALES							
Wash., D.C.	87	46	73	10	0	34	24
San Diego	83	54	41	36	45	19	2
Philadelphia	80	24	74	12	0	12	—
New York	78	28	72	4	2	16	2
Kansas City	73	24	61	21	2	6	3
Portland	69	33	50	22	11	26	0
New Orleans	65	30	56	22	0	6	6
St. Louis	53	25	39	13	0	4	20
Indianapolis	47	15	30	20	0	6	0
San Antonio	45	25	24	16	3	20	1
Dallas	44	18	34	14	7	5	0

Source: National Institute of Justice/Drug Use Forecasting Program

At one point, people in Miami told me that crack-related violence had become so severe that they were afraid to even honk their horns while driving. They were afraid the other driver was so hopped up he'd fire a gun or try to run them off the road. One reason cocaine use among professional football players came to light is that nonusing players were terrified of the violent fury that the drug could cause. As one player told me, he'd look across the line and see the opponent—his pupils huge, his face a slab of raw fury—and he'd know he was in deep trouble. The violent behavior of crack users has even made it difficult for emergency medical personnel to help overdose victims. In schools across the nation, incidents of violence are on the rise, due in no small part to drugs. As one principal told me, "If you so much as ask a student the time of day, you risk having a knife pulled on you."

Crack Babies

Another social side effect is the tragedy of babies born addicted to crack. In some areas, up to 27 percent of newborns have cocaine in their bodies at the time of delivery. These poor kids come into the world with severe physical and mental abnormalities. Because cocaine narrows their mothers' blood vessels, they had a reduced supply of oxygen in the womb, which can thwart development. Also, a breakdown product of cocaine gets trapped in the mother's circulation and continues to hammer away at the fetus's heart and brain, leading to neurological changes that the kid may not grow out of. If a cocaine-using mother insists on breast-feeding her newborn, she continues to pass the drug to the kid in her milk.

If you observe a crack baby in the days after delivery, you notice he's not like the other kids. He is stiff and tense; his cries are piercing and panicky. It's as if every nerve in his body is firing all at once. Close to 20 percent of these babies have abnormal EEG readings and many have patches of dead tissue in their brains. They are three times as likely to die of sudden infant death syndrome (SIDS) than babies born to heroin addicts. Those who do survive are likely to experience visual impairments, mental retardation, delayed development, symptoms of stroke, and learning problems.

We have evidence now that these kids are born with a form

of minimal brain dysfunction and are more likely to become hyperactive and to have difficulty focusing in school. If the infant survives, it will likely suffer a lifelong difficulty in succeeding.

Very important work by pediatrician Ira Chasnoff has shown that crack is giving birth to a whole new generation of people who suffer debilitating problems before they even see the light of day.

Cocaine, marijuana, and alcohol are the Top Three Hits on today's substance abuse charts. But as we'll see in the next chapter, some golden oldies, including LSD, are making a comeback. And some brand new contenders have made the list with a bullet.

CHAPTER EIGHT

Ecstasy, Ice, and Others: More Drug Battles to Be Won

Deep down, I truly believe that we will win the war against drugs. I admit, though, that sometimes it seems like the road to victory gets longer every day. Drugs are like the mythological multiheaded Hydra—chop off one of its heads and two more emerge. One day the statistics show we are making tremendous progress against marijuana and cocaine. The next day we read that drug dealers have come up with an even deadlier creation. Today anyone with a dime-store chemistry set and a recipe can synthesize pure, concentrated hell in a test tube.

In this chapter I'll describe some drugs of recent vintage, as well as some that are based on substances people have been abusing for thousands of years.

Ice

To the Japanese, it's *shabu.* To Koreans, it's *hiroppon.* To Filipinos, it's *batu.*

To Americans, it's ice.

"Ice" is crystallized methamphetamine, a smokable and

more powerful version of amphetamine—speed—that resembles fragments of glass, rock candy, salt, or ice chips. Over the years other drugs, including crack, have been called ice in some locales; today, though, ice has come to mean crystal methamphetamine exclusively.

No one knows when ice first appeared, but methamphetamine itself isn't anything new. It was cooked up by a Japanese chemist in the late 1800s. During World War II, Japanese military leaders gave the drug to their soldiers and to people working in munitions plants to keep them alert and productive. After the war many workers continued using speed, still a legal drug, as they struggled to rebuild their nation. Today, while use has tapered off, there are still close to half a million methamphetamine addicts in Japan, making it that country's number one drug of abuse.

Ice is just methamphetamine in crystal rock form; speed is also available in pills or powder (called "crank" in some places), and as an injectable solution.

In the summer of 1988, use of ice became widespread in Hawaii, probably because of its proximity to the Far East and because crack had gotten so much publicity. You know the kind of thinking: "Hey, you want a smokable drug that looks like little rocks and really gets you off? Crack is for wimps. *This* is the real thing!" Within a year ice surpassed marijuana and cocaine as the islands' biggest drug problem.

Most ice is imported from Asia, but drug dealers in this country are learning how to make it domestically. Ice sells for about $40,000 a pound wholesale. On the street, users can buy about one tenth of a gram for $50. This dose, which can come in a plastic bag the size of a penny, is sometimes called a "paper." A new user can stay high on this much ice for up to a week. Of course dealers, eager to cash in on the drug's growing popularity, will sell everything from Epsom salts to quartz crystals and call it ice. After all, when buyers find out they've been ripped off, who are they going to complain to? The Better Business Bureau?

A pipe used for smoking ice is different from one used for

crack. It looks like a test tube with a hollow ball at the end. An ice crystal about the size of a grain of rice is dropped into the main chamber and heated. The crystal melts to a liquid, then vaporizes. Ice produces what users call "cool smoke"—clean and white—as opposed to the dirty brown "hot smoke" of crack. Users only need to inhale one or two hits to get high. They then wrap the pipe in a cold towel or paper, which helps the residue to recrystallize, all ready for another dose.

Amphetamine and its varieties stimulate and accelerate the central nervous system—that is, after all, why they call it speed. As with crack smoking, inhaling ice smoke sends a rush of large amounts of the drug to the brain (via the lungs). Intravenous use of methamphetamine means the drug has to float through the bloodstream before reaching the brain.

According to substance abuse expert David Smith, cocaine is in the "minor leagues" compared to ice. Like crack, ice produces its high in less than ten seconds. Some users refer to getting high as "amping," because of the amplified sense of euphoria. Unlike crack, though, the high can last anywhere from eight to 24 *hours.* For users searching for thrills, the thought of such a long-term high is virtually irresistible.

For several reasons—its unique chemical structure and its lower melting point among them—ice may be even more addictive than crack, and the habit may be harder to kick. (One Drug Enforcement Administration official remarked that ice is such a nightmare that he longs for the "good old crack days.") A user can quickly become hooked. Ice can be fatal—we have reports of dozens of deaths, many of them suicides and many of them homicides.

Next to the high, the most dramatic effect of ice is weight loss. Virtually every ice smoker who seeks treatment reports this problem to one degree or another. Prolonged use can cause fatal lung and kidney disorders. A recent report in the Journal of the American Medical Association described the association between smoking ice and the very serious and often fatal heart disease called cardiomyopathy. Other side effects include rapid breathing, accelerated heartbeat, increased body temperature, anxiety, sudden rise in blood pressure, irritability, nervousness, insomnia, nausea, hot flashes, dry mouth, sweating, and palpitations. As with any drug, use can lead to accidents and trauma.

Ice, like crack, provokes users to extreme violence. Police in Honolulu believe that ice is involved in perhaps 70 percent of the spouse-abuse cases they confront. In that city, six or more "ice babies"—infants already addicted to the drug—are born each week.

Ice users who survive to make it to the emergency room usually exhibit extreme paranoia and auditory hallucinations; some become wildly destructive or have complete psychotic breakdowns. These psychiatric symptoms can persist for days, weeks—*and even longer.* Some doctors are working with patients who still can't function nearly three years after they stopped smoking.

Even with the recent media attention and the potential this attention has to stimulate the drug user's curiosity, ice has largely been isolated as a West Coast problem. But as a drug treatment specialist, I must admit that I am extremely concerned that ice might follow the path of crack.

Hallucinogens

Since the day the first humans stood upright, people have sought to alter, control, or expand their consciousness, to find Truth with a capital *T.* Many such seekers believe that the way to open the mind is through chemicals that induce visions. Some of these chemicals can be found in nature—in mushrooms, roots, and herbs. Others are cooked up in basement laboratories. Regardless of their source, these drugs change the way users perceive the world and their place within it, changes that aren't necessarily for the better.

Although we're not sure how they work, these drugs produce hallucinations: abnormal sensory feelings that arise without any stimulation from outside one's body. An auditory hallucination, for example, means that a person hears voices when no one is speaking. Any of the five senses—taste, touch, sight, smell, hearing—can succumb to hallucinations. For some reason, many of these feelings are perceived by the body as visual signals. People zonked on hallucinogens may "see" music or believe they see insects crawling on the wallpaper.

Hallucinogens were all the rage a couple of decades ago. Lately they've enjoyed a resurgence. Let's look at some of the more common forms of these drugs.

LSD: Invented by a Swiss scientist named Albert Hoffmann, LSD—lysergic acid diethylamide—is the most notorious of the hallucinogens. It rose to prominence in the 1960s, when it became an ingrained part of the countercultural revolution. Harvard professor Timothy Leary made a name for himself by advocating use of this drug and running around the country urging kids to "tune in, turn on, drop out." As I mentioned earlier, LSD, along with marijuana, may be making a comeback with some affluent suburban teenagers obsessed with capturing 1960s nostalgia.

LSD, or "acid," is colorless, tasteless, and odorless, and comes in different forms: "blotter," or tiny squares of colored paper in which a drop of the drug has been absorbed; "window pane," a clear gelatin form; or in a pill. Many a college student began his first "trip" by sucking on a sugar cube laced with LSD.

The high kicks in within a half hour or so. Users report a kaleidoscopic array of colors, sights, and sounds. Time seems to stand still. Space distorts; one patient told me she was tripping while riding a bicycle, and the road under her wheels seemed to stretch and contract in a rhythmic, pulsating movement.

For some, the experience of having their senses assaulted and battered seems vastly entertaining. For others, it is infinitely frightening—a "bad trip," in the lingo of the user. The hallucinogenic effects of LSD mimic symptoms of schizophrenia: hearing voices, seeing things that aren't there, and having a creepy, paranoid feeling that everything is wildly out of whack. While the sensory roller coaster ride might last two or three hours, the schizophrenic effects might persist half a day or more. Many users report "flashbacks"—LSD effects that recur spontaneously months after the drug was used.

LSD isn't very addicting; few people become tolerant of its

effects or develop dependency. Bad trips, however, have caused many cases of permanent psychosis and have driven some users to suicide. There are published reports of users who hallucinated that they had extraordinary powers, such as the ability to fly, and who killed themselves by jumping out of windows or off mountains.

Mescaline (peyote): Mescaline is the psychoactive substance found in the "buttons" on peyote cactuses. These "buttons" are dried and eaten or mixed in tea. Pure mescaline can be taken in capsules or dissolved in water and swallowed. Mescaline and peyote have similar psychedelic effects, but peyote seems to be stronger, possibly because it contains other drugs as well. Aldous Huxley, who wrote *Brave New World,* experimented with mescaline in the 1950s, and peyote is mentioned frequently in the "Don Juan" books by Carlos Castaneda. Some Indian tribes continue to use peyote in their religious rituals, an act permitted by U.S. law. Peyote and mescaline produce a high that is milder than the one from LSD and that leaves one's sense of self relatively intact. However, they often cause nausea and vomiting. They also may produce flashbacks and can trigger psychological problems.

Psilocybin: This is the active substance found in the nearly 80 varieties of "magic mushrooms" that grow all over the world. Use of mushrooms in Mexico dates as far back as 1,000 years before the Christian era. Mushrooms can be eaten raw, cooked into recipes, or brewed as a tea; the powder containing the psilocybin can be eaten, snorted, or taken in a capsule. The effects of these "shrooms," similar to LSD and peyote but milder, usually peak after about 90 minutes. The more mushrooms one eats, the longer the high lasts. Psilocybin can cause anxiety, depression, disorientation, and loss of touch with reality. Some people get sick because they eat poisonous mushrooms thinking, wrongly, that they contain psilocybin.

Dimethyltryptamine (DMT): Similar to psilocybin, this drug occurs naturally in a spruce plant native to parts of South America and the West Indies. It can also be synthesized in a test tube. DMT usually shows up in powder form that is mixed as a liquid, soaked onto tobacco, marijuana, even parsley, and smoked. It can also be swallowed or injected. The effects of DMT, which are similar to those of LSD, may last no more than half an hour.

STP: This synthetic hallucinogen, a form of amphetamine, gets its name from the gasoline additive marketed as a way to improve engine performance. STP, a relative of Ecstasy (see below), combines the hallucinations of LSD with the speeding effects of amphetamines. Although widely used for a while, STP lost popularity because its effects last so long—ebbing and flowing—that many users feel their trip will never end.

Designer Drugs

Chemicals are like Tinkertoys. With a little fiddling, you can stick a doohickey here, attach a thingamabob there and—voilà! A brand new whatchamacallit.

People who make designer drugs take a chemical, change it just a little, and sell it as something entirely new. These people aren't exactly motivated by the search for, say, a cancer cure. What they're doing is taking an illegal or controlled substance and turning it into something that never existed before. These new drugs are thus legal—or, more accurately, they are not yet illegal. Even if a drug is eventually placed on the restricted list, all the chemist has to do is tinker with it some more, change the name, and he's back in action. This back-alley enterprise—a blend of chemistry and crime—has burgeoned into a billion-dollar business.

Designer drugs have been around for decades; their roots go back to the chemists who whipped up batches of LSD and other such drugs. Crack, in fact, is a kind of designer cocaine, developed through experiments by "street chemists" who were looking for a safer way to freebase. Most designer drugs available today are variations on the old themes: narcotics, stimulants, painkillers, or hallucinogens.

PCP: First synthesized by researchers as an anesthetic in

1958, PCP (phencyclidine) is a highly dangerous drug with a variety of names: angel dust, peace, Captain Crunch. It can be eaten, injected, snorted, or mixed with marijuana and smoked as "superweed."

In early clinical tests, PCP caused people to become overexcited after an operation and produced fearful delusions and psychotic behavior. No wonder doctors decided the drug had no place in medicine. But that didn't stop it from filtering out into the street, where it first appeared in San Francisco in 1967. For a while PCP was a "drug of deception"—that is, it was sold to unsuspecting buyers as LSD or as "pure THC" in capsule form. Soon, though, users came to feel that PCP had virtues of its own.

The effects of PCP are unpredictable and frightening. One problem is that PCP works as an anesthetic while stimulating the muscles. Users may thus do risky things but are unable to feel the pain that would normally warn them of danger. There are cases of people high on PCP who have been badly burned or bruised, or who have suffered broken bones, without being aware of the pain—until the drug wore off. For some reason, many PCP users seem attracted to water, and will try to swim even if they don't know how; drowning while on PCP is common. Other effects include sweating, flushing, pronounced drooling, constricted pupils, dizziness, and slurred speech. Because the body takes so long to eliminate the drug, users may experience flashbacks weeks after taking PCP.

Acute poisoning by PCP makes people violent, or induces convulsions, catatonia, and coma—sometimes within minutes of taking the dose. In some cases, the drug produces fatal increases in blood pressure. Some users "moon walk"—they act as if they're trying to walk on the moon in a space suit. Repeated use of high doses can produce impaired judgment, paranoid delusions, hallucinations, and destructive behavior, which may last for as long as a week. Some users suffer psychotic episodes that last a month or more, even after taking a single dose. Chronic users are at risk of depression that can lead to suicide.

The negative publicity PCP received in the 1970s led us to

hope that the drug would disappear. Lately, though, it seems to have enjoyed a dismaying revival in popularity. Up to a third of patients involuntarily entering psychiatric hospitals admitted to being PCP users. There's no evidence that PCP is physically addictive, but long-term use may create tolerance and, as I've shown, can result in severe psychological problems.

Users call PCP angel dust—I call it devil's dirt.

Ecstasy: This so-called "wonder drug" with the Madison Avenue name received a lot of publicity in the mid-1980s—even appearing on the cover of *New York* magazine—an issue that I still find hard to believe. Because it produces a feeling of well-being, comfort, and confidence, it was touted as "the love drug" and was used experimentally as an adjunct to psychotherapy, especially for couples. Some therapists believed that patients who used this drug would be more open and honest with each other. But the therapeutic value of the drug has never been proved.

Ecstasy belongs to the family of drugs known as methoxylated amphetamines—amphetamines dressed up with ribbons and bows to make them a cross between a stimulant and a hallucinogen, similar to STP. Strictly speaking, Ecstasy is methylenedioxymethamphetamine, or MDMA, but similar compounds, such as MDA and MMDA, are also sold under the same name.

The popularity of Ecstasy followed the typical pattern: publicity in the media, leading to use by celebrities, followed by claims of safety in the absence of valid scientific research. Then, however, the *Journal of the American Medical Association* reported five deaths in the Dallas, Texas, area that were attributed to Ecstasy. Use tapered off, especially after the DEA placed the drug on its list of controlled substances.

Users of these amphetamine derivatives report feeling a warm glow that spreads through their bodies, followed by a sense of physical and mental well-being that intensifies gradually and steadily. For some people, Ecstasy produces feelings reported by users as delight, empathy, serenity, joy, insight, and self-awareness but without hallucinations or a feeling that one is out of control. Unlike most stimulants, MDA suppresses motor activity, rather than increasing it.

However, as with any psychedelic drug, there are dangers. MDA saps the user's energy. It can reactivate infections, especially in the urinary tract. It produces tension in the muscles of the face and jaw, which may lead to involuntary teeth grinding or jerky eye movements. Some users report intense anxiety, panic, or paranoid reactions. Others take higher doses or have less resistance to the drug—and report even greater reactions. Some people experience toxic reactions ranging from skin problems, sweating, and confusion to elevated blood pressure, inability to use or understand spoken or written language, brain damage, and death.

Ecstasy? You got to be kidding.

Other Designer Drugs: Recently there appeared to be an outbreak of Parkinson's disease in Northern California. It turns out that a drug designer had altered a narcotic analgesic called fentanyl and produced an analogue called MPTP. One of MPTP's effects is to trigger brain cell damage, paralysis, and the symptoms of Parkinson's—tremor, drooling, difficulty walking, muscle weakness, and emotional instability. Ironically, MPTP is a legal substance commonly used in the chemical industry. Thus, although the drug dealer caused harm to over 400 people, he couldn't be prosecuted for selling an illegal substance. The DEA now has the power to list such new drugs as controlled substances for an emergency period of one year. But that often just means that drug designers get to work, shuffle the molecules in a compound, and come up with something new.

A similar drug, called MPPP (with the catchy name of 1-methyl-4-phenylproionoxypiperidine), is an analogue of meperidine (brand name: Demerol) that is widely available on the West Coast. Officials estimate that perhaps 20 percent of California's 200,000 heroin addicts now use MPPP. While fentanyl is highly addictive and is a hundred times more powerful than morphine, MPPP is thought to be *2,000 times* more powerful than morphine. MPPP has been linked to over 100 deaths on the West Coast. The amount of this drug needed to supply the entire country could be made in a single lab in just one week and stored in a shoebox. One recent study revealed that a single drop of pure MPPP could kill 50 people. Yet another form of fentanyl, known as "China White," is sold as a kind of heroin.

The final word on designer drugs will probably never be written. As long as people turn outside themselves to drugs, in their search for happiness, excitement, or cosmic vision, crooks posing as chemists will thrive. True scientists, however, don't create drugs for fun; they do so to relieve suffering and conquer disease. In the long history of substance abuse, no single designer drug has ever been shown to help anybody—except, perhaps, the con artists who cook them up.

Heroin and Methadone

For decades heroin was the main drug of addiction. Today it has been eclipsed by cocaine, especially crack. But it's still with us, and still a significant problem. Heroin use may be increasing as cocaine and crack addicts attempt to calm down. There are perhaps 700,000 heroin addicts in the United States. New addicts seem to appear as fast as others are treated or die from an overdose or AIDS.

Unlike some of the designer drugs, which spring up overnight and sometimes fade just as quickly, heroin has a long history. For centuries humans have used opium—the sap that oozes from poppies. In 1806, a scientist isolated morphine, the active ingredient in opium, which gets its name from Morpheus, the Greek god of dreams. Nearly 70 years later an English research chemist created an artificial morphine, and by 1898 this product was marketed by Bayer, the German pharmaceutical maker, under the brand name of Heroin.

At first, heroin was seen to hold great promise as a treatment for pain, for cough and other respiratory ailments, and as a "nonaddicting" substitute for morphine. Even today, it still has its advocates as an analgesic. Many tonics and nostrums available at the turn of the century contained bizarre combinations of heroin, cocaine, and other addicting substances.

Soon heroin became a street drug especially popular among

the poor and minorities. As usual, the experts were late to respond. Finally, in the early 1900s heroin was made illegal.

In the late 1960s heroin addiction emerged as a problem connected to the counterculture movement. The new heroin addict was now white and middle class, compared to the poor black addicts of previous decades. Many American GIs in Vietnam turned to heroin—there was plenty of it around and it was capable of creating a dreamlike diversion from war. In recent years, abuse of heroin has sprung up among a new demographic group: some well-off overachievers and others who prefer high-purity "Persian" heroin, heroin when it's mixed with cocaine freebase. Some users manage to "chip"—that is, they use the drug occasionally, living somewhat normal lives, complete with jobs and families. Today heroin is usually smuggled into this country as part of shipments of furniture or rugs from Asia. Some even arrives sewn into the bodies of live goldfish.

Heroin is a white, bitter-tasting powder. Users liquefy the powder by cooking it, usually on a bent spoon held over a candle or other flame, and inject it. Heroin can be snorted, but the IV route gives a more intense rush and is more quickly addicting. Purity is a problem; samples of heroin from the street range from being a mere 2 percent pure heroin to the 92 percent purity of the Persian variety. The latest craze is heroin in the form called "Mexican tar" or "tootsie roll," which is a dark, gummy version of relatively high potency.

The first effect users of heroin feel is usually unpleasant, including nausea, sweating, and discomfort. Eventually, though, users experience a rush of good feeling, followed by the "nod," a period of relaxation and drowsiness.

It's easy to take a fatal overdose of heroin, especially given the wild fluctuations in purity and the user's increasing level of tolerance, which always progresses toward the lethal dose. And heroin is highly addictive. Users pass quickly through the stages of tolerance and dependency; those who try to quit suffer severe physical withdrawal symptoms. It is, in fact, the interaction between the euphoric rush and the fear of withdrawal that compels users to keep shooting up.

Like cocaine, heroin becomes more important than anything else, including sex. Although a single dose of heroin may be relatively cheap, addicts need so much of the drug that they often turn to crime—theft, blackmail, prostitution—to support their habits. They have to find it, get it ready, and use it so many times in a day that their life becomes a constant cycle of "craving-seeking-use." And as you are no doubt aware, the biggest risk factor today for the spread of AIDS comes from addicts, particularly heroin addicts, who share needles. Users are also prone to malnutrition, problems with blood circulation, constipation, and tuberculosis. Pregnant women who use heroin cause their babies to be born addicted and to suffer the agonies of withdrawal in their first days of life.

For a quarter of a century, pharmacological treatment for heroin addiction relied on methadone, a synthetic opiate developed by German scientists during World War II. In the 1960s Methadone began to be used as a way to detoxify addicts and help them maintain a heroin-free life. Methadone replaces the extreme craving for heroin but with less sedation, thus helping addicts live a more normal life at less risk. The plan is usually to gradually withdraw the methadone and help the patient become completely drug-free. Others stay on methadone maintenance of one dose per day. They are freed of needles, craving, and seeking—many are able to get and hold jobs for the first time. Ironically, though, methadone has become a substance of abuse on its own, and is often stolen from clinics and sold as a street drug.

Part of the good news is that a medication called clonidine (sold as Catapres) offers the first nonaddictive, nonnarcotic treatment for opiate withdrawal—a treatment that was invented by my colleagues and I at Yale University. Clonidine "fools" the brain into thinking it's not in withdrawal, when in fact it is. With this drug, an addict can be free of opiate dependency in less than two weeks. Use of naltrexone (another treatment that my colleagues and I pioneered) then helps maintain the drug-free state. Naltrexone (brand name: Trexan) fits into the same receptors in the brain that heroin and methadone do, thus blocking the effects of opiates. If a patient taking naltrexone shoots up, the heroin will circulate in the bloodstream like a car looking for a parking space in a crowded lot. Eventually the heroin is excreted without having the chance to produce its effects. Like clonidine, it was obvious to doctors and patients alike that naltrexone was a medication that worked from the very first day.

Incidentally, it is very gratifying to find that our discovery of clonidine efficacy enables babies born addicted to heroin to be detoxified. Also, our patients appreciate DuPont's producing naltrexone in pill form (in the early days it was administered in a rather noxious, slimy liquid).

Prescription Drugs

I could make a strong case that the most abused drugs in the country today are ones that are perfectly legal and supplied, not by your traditional drug dealers, but by your friendly neighborhood doctors and pharmacists. Over two billion—that's billion with a *b*—prescriptions are written in this country each year. In most instances, these drugs do the trick: They relieve suffering and rout disease. But when prescribed indiscriminately, or when patients misuse them either deliberately or through misunderstanding, they can be deadly.

The drugs I'm most concerned about are the ones used successfully in psychiatry, my own area of specialty. These drugs are known as *psychoactive* drugs because they work directly in, and on, the brain to change the way it operates. Other drugs, such as antibiotics, go to the site of the problem—say, streptococcus in the throat—and do their work there, by routing invading bacteria or clearing up inflammation. Psychoactive drugs account for only about 20 percent of the medications we use, but their potential for abuse is generally much higher than the remaining 80 percent.

Drugs in this category include tranquilizers, sedatives, narcotic analgesics, antipsychotics, antidepressants, and stimulants (see Box on page 170). These substances circulate to the brain where they produce changes in the electrochemical system that governs the way we think and feel. For example, when the body suffers pain, cells release chemicals that trigger electrical responses alerting the brain that there's a problem. A painkilling drug, however, attaches itself to the receptors on certain nerves, blocking the chemical messengers and preventing them from triggering that pain response. Other psychoactive drugs affect other neurotransmitter systems, including the ones that regulate mood and appetite. Some drugs, which work just the way the body's own neurotransmitters do, act to block these systems, give them a "jump start," or increase their capacity to function.

Strangely, no one—including the people who invented them—actually knows how these drugs work. That's one thing that makes them so dangerous. We don't completely understand all their actions. And most drugs do more than one thing. Amphetamines are used in diet pills because they decrease appetite, but they also speed up the entire nervous system (although they slow down hyperactive children and improve their concentration). Antidepressants alter the mood of a person with clinical depression, but they also affect the heart, blood pressure, digestion, and sexual appetite. Besides depression, antidepressants may also be used to treat panic attacks and even bed-wetting. In prescribing these medications, doctors must consider both benefit and risk; if the former doesn't outweigh the latter, the drug shouldn't be used.

Medications can save lives, but they can also pose a serious risk of abuse. Some have a greater addiction potential than others, but many of them, taken in high enough doses for long enough periods, produce tolerance, leading to dependency. Valium, for example, was for many years considered a "minor" tranquilizer; recently, over 60 million prescriptions for Valium were written. Valium may be a "wonder drug," but we now know that this and other drugs in its class (the benzodiazepines) can be highly addicting—there's nothing "minor" about them. Recently New York State changed its laws and required

Psychoactive Drugs

Sedative Hypnotics

Purpose: Relief of tension, improved sleep

Examples: Nembutal (phenobarbital), Placidyl (ethchlorvynol), Seconal (secobarbital)

Narcotic Analgesics

Purpose: Relief of pain

Examples: Darvon (propoxyphene), Demerol (meperidine), Dilaudid (hydromorphone)

Stimulants

Purpose: Increase alertness, energy

Examples: Cylert (pemoline), Dexedrine (dextroamphetamine), Ritalin (methylphenidate)

Tranquilizers

Purpose: Relief of minor tension and anxiety

Examples: Librium (chlordiazepoxide hydrochloride), Valium (diazepam), Xanax (alprazolam)

Antidepressants

Purpose: Relief of depression

Examples: Elavil (amitriptyline), Sinequan (doxepin), Tofranil (imipramine), Prozac (fluoxetine)

Antipsychotics

Purpose: Control major mental illness, such as schizophrenia

Examples: Compazine (prochlorperazine), Haldol (haloperidol), Thorazine (chlorpromazine)

doctors to report all prescriptions for Valium in the same way they must report prescriptions for barbiturates. Xanax, a benzodiazepine–like medication, is even more popular than Valium. Unfortunately, Xanax can be very addicting, making a patient's withdrawal very difficult. Researchers are currently working on new medications that may someday greatly reduce the benzodiazepine's addiction potential.

These drugs are, and will remain, valuable weapons in the fight against psychiatric illness. They have saved hundreds of thousands of lives, and have improved the outlook for millions of people. But they are nonetheless dangerous and powerful chemicals, and they must be handled with extreme care.

The good news is that public awareness of this problem has risen enormously in just the past few years. We're not the same nation of people who, a few decades ago, thought we could swallow a pill and make all our problems disappear. As we become increasingly health conscious—a change fueled in part by more and better coverage of medical issues in the media—we no longer grab for the medicine bottle at the first twinge of pain or unhappiness. As consumers, Americans are demanding more information about their prescriptions from their doctors, and will seek a second opinion if they don't think taking a powerful and dangerous drug is the right thing to do.

And that's a change in the right direction.

CHAPTER NINE

The Weapons We Need . . . In Our Homes

Like charity, the fight against drug use begins at home. When I'm asked to name the most important weapon we have against drugs, I do not hesitate: The answer is "Parents." No other antidrug strategy—interdiction, treatment, punishment—works as well as good old parenting.

Children inherit more than just blue eyes or a button nose from their parents. They also inherit a system of values. They see and interpret the world through a parent's eyes. They develop their moral compass, the instinctive sense of the right thing to do, by observing their parents' behavior and beliefs.

Parents naturally try to protect their children from harm. They keep them from tumbling down the basement stairs or from touching hot stoves. By the same token, they can show their children how to keep from getting burned by drugs—*if* they know that doing so is a vital part of their responsibility and *if* they learn the right techniques.

Briefly stated, those techniques are: Learn the facts about drugs and drug abuse. Realize the impact your own attitudes will have on your child. Understand young people's attitudes and the other factors that may lead them to experiment with these substances. Recognize the signs of abuse. Most important, know when and how to intervene.

By reading the first half of this book, you're already accomplished the first step of learning the facts. I encourage you to continue your education by reading more and talking with other parents, doctors, and drug experts. Getting involved with school and local drug programs will keep you abreast of developments in your community. The drug abuse picture in this country changes virtually every week, as new drugs and new methods of abuse emerge with alarming regularity.

Attitudes

Not long ago we talked with a patient named Romain who wanted desperately to kick his crack habit. Since working with the family is a critical part of treatment, we arranged to meet with the boy's mother. Within minutes of meeting her we learned the true source of Romain's problem. You see, the mother had actually encouraged her son to quit school and set up shop as a cocaine dealer. Access to the drug had only made Romain's own drug habit much worse. "I know you think I'm terrible," said the mother. "But let me tell you something: Since his father died we don't have enough money for rent, let alone food. You show me another way we can bring in $500 a week, and I'll be happy to send Romain back to school." Later, Romain echoed this theme when he said that, as the "man of the family," it had fallen on him to put bread on the table, and he did so in the only way that was open to him.

Prevention starts with the family. Parents who demonstrate the right attitudes about drugs—not just illicit drugs but also about alcohol, cigarettes, even caffeine and prescription medications—eliminate the biggest single risk factor for drug abuse.

Of course, it's hard for parents to show a kid what the right attitude is if they themselves are substance abusers, or confused about drugs. The reddest of red flags warning of danger is that one or both parents suffer from chemical dependency or some other form of compulsive or addictive disorder. Parents who deal with their problems by drinking or using drugs send a clear, but wrong, signal to their children: "This is the way to handle stress."

In a survey we conducted through the 800-COCAINE helpline, 41 percent of callers said their parents used marijuana or other drugs, although these same parents claimed that they disapproved of drug use by adolescents. This attitude—"do as I say, not as I do"—just doesn't wash when it comes to preventing drug use. If these parents had suited their words to their actions, our helpline would have a lot fewer calls to deal with—and that would be just fine with me.

The parental drug of abuse can even be as seemingly innocuous as nicotine or caffeine. If a parent drinks coffee compulsively, a child will tend to accept *all* kinds of compulsive behavior as normal. And parents who use tobacco send a "smoke signal" that cigarettes are okay. But smoking is nothing more than a drug delivery system, a route by which chemicals enter the body. As I've shown, learning to smoke cigarettes opens the gateway to using other kinds of smokable drugs, including marijuana and crack.

Surveys for the Partnership for a Drug-Free America, conducted in 1987 by the Gordon S. Black Corporation, revealed some astonishing things about the way parents perceive the drug problem:

• *Fifty-one percent of parents think their kids have never used drugs and never will.* Think of it—half of the parents believe, naively, that a drug problem can't happen in their own backyard. Naturally, parents with this attitude don't feel too motivated to work with their children to prevent drug abuse. It's strange: Even though parents think their own children are immune, over 60 percent report that drugs have affected other children they know.

• *More than three in ten parents believe their kids have never been exposed to drugs.* One of my patients said that, during a visit home from college, her parents asked if she smoked marijuana. She said yes, thinking they would be devastated but that they should know the truth. "It was so strange, though," she recalled. "The next time I visited, they asked the exact same question, as if they'd never heard my answer! I guess they were so shocked that they couldn't absorb what I was telling them. They wanted so desperately to believe their little girl was still 'pure' that they just blocked out anything they didn't want to hear."

• *A large group—43 percent—think their children don't have the money to buy drugs.* Apparently, these parents are unaware that a vial of crack costs as much as a couple of *Batman* comic books, or that a joint of marijuana goes for the same price as a premium ice cream bar. If their allowances are inadequate, or if they happen to spend their lunch money on lunch, young drug users will steal from parents or friends in their search for the next high.

• *Nearly three out of ten parents said cigarettes were worse than pot.* These parents need to learn the facts: that marijuana smoke contains cancer-causing compounds, that the THC content of the dope available today is much higher than dope of their generation, and that the method of smoking—inhaling deeply and holding in the smoke as long as possible—makes one joint just as dangerous as a whole pack of cigarettes. And, contrary to previous belief, marijuana is addicting.

• *More than one adult in four thinks it's okay to smoke pot in private.* Smoking in the privacy of your own bedroom doesn't make it any less dangerous to your health than toking up at a rock concert.

• *One in five adults sees cocaine as a status symbol.* Parents with this attitude are what I call snow-blind—they have fallen for the myth that coke is the "success drug," used by people with money and influence. I wish I could take these parents on a 15-second tour of a crack house. If they could see the squalor and degradation, they'd whistle a different tune about the "status" cocaine conveys on its victims.

• *Eleven percent feel that occasional use of cocaine is not risky.* Wrong. Onetime use of cocaine can lead to addiction, health problems, even death.

My point is simply that parents' attitudes—right or wrong—are passed on to children. Earlier, in our discussion of addiction, I stated that drug use leads to physical tolerance. In a sense, the reverse is true: Tolerance—and here I mean the attitude of tolerance—leads to drug use.

The good news is that the situation is changing. In its follow-up survey, conducted in 1989, the Gordon S. Black Corporation noted that parents are becoming much more sensitized to the dangers of drug use, and that attitudes toward drugs are becoming "distinctly more antagonistic." The same is true among all age groups, especially among college students. Seven out of ten parents report that they have taken the time to discuss the problem of drug use with their children, and have taken an antidrug stand. More than three out of ten state that they have gone so far as to discuss the problem with parents of other children whom they know to be using drugs. That sort of report brings a smile to my face.

Let's look at the subject of attitudes from the adolescent's point of view.

Almost half of the teenagers who use marijuana regularly fear that they will get caught by the law. An even greater number fear getting caught by parents or school authorities. Parents can exploit these fearful attitudes in constructive ways. They can teach their children that there is good reason to fear the law: Marijuana is illegal everywhere in the country. Parents can learn about the penalties for drug use in their own state and communities, and share these facts with their children. A kid who finds out that getting caught with a bag of marijuana in the car can automatically land him in jail will be less inclined to use the drug.

Likewise, parents should learn what their school's policy about drug use is and reinforce that policy in the home. If a child learns, for example, that the parents will report his drug use to school authorities, he will certainly be less inclined to experiment.

Roughly four out of ten adolescents fear that their own drug use will negatively influence their siblings. Again, a reasonable fear, since younger brothers and sisters do look up to older ones as role models and are extremely influenced by them. Parents can hammer home the message that older children bear a responsibility to protect their younger siblings by setting a good example.

One teenager in three is afraid of getting hold of impure marijuana; twice that number fear impure cocaine or crack. Parents can reinforce the point that street drugs are notoriously —and perhaps lethally—full of impurities. Laboratory analysis has from time to time turned up samples of marijuana tainted with herbicides, insecticides, LSD, amphetamines, strychnine—even rat poison. Heroin may be only 2 percent pure. Cocaine may be laced with anything from baking soda to quinine to Drano; contrary to myth, the crack form of cocaine isn't "pure" cocaine—crack only concentrates any impurities that were in the original cocaine powder.

Close to 30 percent of those surveyed were concerned that drugs will affect their performance in school. They're absolutely right. As we've seen, drugs wipe out short-term memory, rob kids of motivation, and ruin concentration. Parents should calmly get this message across. Most adolescents are so focused on the "here and now" that they can't think in terms of the future. Thus it probably does little good to try and explain that drug use today might keep kids from being accepted at the college of their choice, or from pursuing the career of their dreams—but those are certainly likely scenarios.

Nearly six out of ten teenagers fear that cocaine use will lead to physical or psychological damage; half of them fear becoming dependent on the drug. Parents who realize that these fears are completely justified can make the point in a loving yet firm way, and in so doing steer their children away from a lifetime of misery.

Parents whose own antidrug attitudes are firmly established are in good shape to steer their children safely through the treacherous waters of adolescence. Other parents may need help in developing these attitudes. Thus, on every level, drug prevention programs should teach parents their children are at

Predisposing Factors of Drug Abuse

Parental alcohol or drug problems
Divorce, money problems, or other sources of family stress
Perceived use of drugs by siblings or friends
Poor parent-child communication
Access to illicit drugs
Preexisting psychological or behavioral problems
Extensive peer involvement with drugs

(Adapted from Mark S. Gold, M.D., *Marijuana*, New York: Plenum Medical Book Company, 1989, p. 207. Used by permission.)

high risk of early drug use and show how to recognize the warning signals. Many teenagers think the behavior of drug users is stupid; the wise parent picks up on that theme and emphasizes it, along with the fact that society on the whole disapproves of drug use. Parents who learn to exploit the child's fears of getting caught, of using impure drugs, or of possible harm to their bodies and brains do better than if they lean too heavily on the old "doom, despair, and death" theme. And parents who can and do talk to their children about drugs—early and often—are rewarded.

Other Risk Factors

When parents have solid antidrug attitudes, backed up by a firm grasp of the facts about drugs, they have laid the foundation for a drug-free life for their children. However, they must also be aware of the other risk factors that can lead to drug abuse. A list of these factors appears in the Box above. A young person at particular risk is one who has a low sense of self-esteem, whose skills at dealing with other people are below par, who has trouble coping with society and its institutions, who has trouble making and keeping friends, or whose family relationships are impaired.

These factors do not *cause* drug abuse, but they suggest

underlying problems that may influence someone to experiment with drugs. For example, a teenager may be suffering from an undiagnosed psychiatric illness such as clinical depression. As a consequence her grades may drop suddenly. In an attempt to self-medicate her depression, this young woman may feel compelled to turn to drugs.

Likewise, a poor relationship between parents, or between parents and children, complicates the picture enormously. As one patient told me, "Why should I talk to my parents about drugs? We don't even talk about who I'm dating." When the lines of communication among family members have been cut, it can take a great effort to restore them. But doing so is necessary for everyone's health, not just the one who's abusing drugs.

Show me a family in which an older sibling uses drugs, and I'll show you a family that needs instant attention. Surveys reveal that children between the ages of nine and 12 who have a drug-abusing older brother or sister are nine times more likely to use marijuana than other children. Older children fail to realize the extent to which their younger siblings will spy on them, and have no conception of the harm their drug use can do to the family as a whole. As Gordon Black observes, older siblings are role models whether they like it or not: "If they can be persuaded to 'turn off,' we can reduce dramatically the likelihood that their brothers and sisters will 'turn on.' "

Second only to sibling influence is peer influence. The simple act of talking with friends about drugs raises the risk. So much of adolescents' identities are tied up with those of their friends that they imitate each other, sometimes to a ridiculous degree. Kids find it hard to say no to their friends. Add the fact that most young people are notoriously ill-informed about the dangers of drugs, and that they perceive drug users as being "cool" and "having lots of friends," and you have a formula for disaster. As Black's surveys conclude, all present and future drug use among teenagers is related to having friends who also use drugs. Children whose friends use pot are eight times more likely to try the drug than other children.

As the report on President Bush's National Drug Control Strategy states:

> . . . Notwithstanding popular mythology about shadowy, raincoated pushers corrupting young innocents on school playgrounds, children almost never *purchase* their first drug experience. . . . Dealers . . . prefer to avoid the risk of selling their wares to strangers, however young. Similarly, new and novice users themselves are typically reluctant to accept an unfamiliar substance from an unfamiliar face. In fact, young people rarely make *any* independent effort to seek out drugs for the first time. They don't have to; use ordinarily begins through simple personal contact with other users. . . . And so first use invariably involves the free and enthusiastic offer of a drug by a friend.

David Ruffin, the former lead singer for the Temptations, revealed to an interviewer just how hard it is to resist pressure from friends to use drugs. After he completed a four-week treatment program for cocaine abuse, he told his friends to stop using cocaine around him and to refrain from offering him the drug. The result? "Mostly I'm alone now, by myself," he remarked. "I walk into a room and everybody walks out. It's hard, but in time you meet people who don't associate with drugs, and there are some friends of mine who won't give me any [drugs] and will threaten anybody who tries."

Parents can help their children by teaching them that *real* friends, like David Ruffin's, are ones who look out for each other's health and safety.

Recognizing Signs of Drug Use

In some cases, despite strong antidrug attitudes and no matter how much the parents try to control other predisposing factors, prevention fails. When it does, kids begin to flirt with drugs. All too often, infatuation becomes fixation.

Then, early detection becomes the key to a quick and effective cure. What are the warning signs of drug use? There are many, and they fall into different categories. All parents must familiarize themselves with these signs, since the earlier we can spot trouble, the less likely a disastrous outcome. Treatment is best when administered early in the illness. (See Box on pages 182–83.)

As you no doubt realize, you need a doctor to recognize some of these telltale clues, such as an enlarged liver. But parents, especially those who are in close communication with the child's teachers, are in the best position to spot other signs of trouble.

Sometimes the less clinical symptoms are the most revealing: changes in friends, loss of interest in former extracurricular activities, drop in grades, changes in dress or mood, resistance to discipline at home or school, flare-ups of temper, increased borrowing of money, shoplifting or stealing money, greater secrecy, or other such subtle behaviors.

Of course a kid who drops out of the track team isn't necessarily turning into a drug addict. But such changes, seen as part of a larger pattern, can mean trouble.

Intervention

Knowing the signs of drug use is important. Even more important, though, is knowing what to do about it.

The word "intervene" means "to come between." That is precisely what parents must do: step between their child and the menace of drugs. Much of what we know today about effective intervention stems from the experience of counselors who work with alcoholics and their families. Part of the good news is that we have a firm grasp on which methods of intervention work, and which may backfire. Ideally intervention takes place early on to prevent the problem altogether, rather than as a means of initiating treatment. And the chances are better if the person is still in contact with the family, for example, or has a

Signs of Drug Use

Physical Signs

- Increased or decreased tolerance for alcohol or drugs
- Red face, red nose
- Bumps and bruises from falling or other accidents
- Puffiness of face, arms, or legs
- Sudden trouble with vision
- Swollen nasal membrane
- Chest problems, such as bronchitis
- Heart problems, such as accelerated heartbeat or heart failure
- Enlarged liver
- Frequent infections
- Digestive problems
- Lingering colds and flu
- High blood pressure
- Signs of bad nutrition
- Tremors
- Blackouts
- Changes in reflexes
- Loss of coordination
- Dizziness
- Slurred speech
- Insomnia
- Impotence
- Craving for sweets
- Loss of appetite

Mental Signs

- Memory loss
- Confusion and slow comprehension
- Anxiety or depression
- Delirium
- Hallucinations

Behavioral Changes

- Increased reliance on drugs
- Suicidal thoughts or behavior
- Violent or abusive behavior

continued

Suspiciousness
Chronic lying
Unusually passive behavior
Increased severity in already existent neurotic symptoms
Rapid mood changes

Social Signs

Family problems
School problems
Declining participation in sports or hobbies
Change in friends
Frequent changes of jobs, lateness, or other job-related problems
Increased legal problems stemming from behavior
Financial difficulties
Car accidents

Adapted from Mark S. Gold, M.D., *The Facts About Drugs and Alcohol,* New York: Bantam Books, 1987. Used by permission.

good job. Intervention *must* take place if an addict's relationship to drugs has grown stronger than any other relationship in his or her life. But intervention works, no matter how hopeless the situation may seem.

The first point I get across to distraught parents who are confronting drug use is that *they need not face the problem alone.* As a result of our growing understanding about drug addiction, physicians, social workers, counselors, and volunteer groups are available to provide the guidance and support they need.

Most parents are naturally concerned that direct confrontation about drug use will alienate their children. They want to avoid hurling accusations, false or otherwise, that would undermine whatever fragile trust they have built up together. For these reasons I advise parents to develop a relationship with their family doctors or general practitioners. Calling a trusted physician is a much safer course, emotionally, than confronting a family member directly. In their conversation, the parents and the doctor can work out a clear and rational approach to the problem.

One early intervention strategy I recommend is annual urine testing. Some civil libertarians often complain that suchurine testing. Some civil libertarians often complain that such tests smack of Big Brotherhood. But I believe that children who know they will be subjected to a regular testing along with their annual pre-school physical are a lot less likely to object to testing. Drug testing, when used with antidrug educational programs and a good family background, can prevent drug use. In turn, children will experience fewer developmental problems, have less trouble in school, encounter fewer family problems related to drug abuse, and be at lower risk for addiction later in life. I'd say these benefits of urine testing for young people far outweigh any risk to their personal freedom.

Similarly, another form of intervention may mean searching the kid's room. A lot of parents draw the line at this, feeling that such an invasion of privacy might make their kid angry or violate their rights. To this I reply: Any parent who suspects his or her child of using drugs has a right—even an obligation—to intervene. Any room, including a child's bedroom, is a part of the parent's home, and no activity that threatens the health of a child should ever be permitted. Remember, using drugs could *kill* your child.

In the world of drug treatment, though, intervention usually means staging a scene in which users are made to face their problem—and the people who are hurt by it. Such interventions must be directed and aggressive. Remember, we are dealing with a life-threatening problem, one that the drug abuser simply cannot control. As my colleague Irl Extein tells parents, "If you wait for a John Belushi to come to you and say, 'Hey, I'm strung out on cocaine and need help,' you will wait until he's dead."

In many cases I advise that someone other than the parent—a physician, for example, or a substance abuse counselor—be delegated to confront an adolescent initially. For one thing, the presence of an objective third party works to defuse a potentially explosive situation. The young person can direct feelings of anger, betrayal, and rebellion toward someone—often a total stranger—who has been trained to handle such emotions, rather than toward the parents, who are suffering their own emotional anguish. The counselor's calm and reassuring presence allows for a more rational discussion of the risks and consequences of drug use and the options for treatment. Also, so many adolescent substance abusers come from dysfunctional families. Working through a counselor may thus be essential, since relationships with parents may be virtually nonexistent.

The most effective confrontations involve what I call "organized coercion." The person in charge, whether a parent or counselor, gets in touch with everyone directly concerned with the young person's problem. They decide in advance which issues need to be discussed, and which should be avoided. They also agree on the form of treatment the drug user needs. Sometimes the participants even assemble to rehearse their comments and offer suggestions to each other on how to proceed. Doing so reduces confusion and turmoil during the actual event.

On the day of the confrontation these people assemble in one room—at the home, in a motel, a church, a doctor's office, wherever there is appropriate and adequate space. I have participated in confrontations in which the youngster's parents, teacher, minister, coach, best friend, girlfriend, siblings, favorite aunt, and boss were all present. The adolescent is brought to the room, usually under some pretense, since he or she would probably not show up for such an occasion voluntarily.

Regardless of how the confrontation is staged, there are certain concrete goals that must be met. First, the adolescent needs to be told that the people present are motivated by love and concern. That message may not sink in, but nonetheless it must be articulated clearly at the very beginning. Second, the adolescent must hear from everybody present exactly how they perceive the problem and how it has affected them personally. The young person must be confronted with hard evidence that his or her ability to function has deteriorated. Next, the people assembled must present a united front in demanding that the teenager enter treatment.

Last, and most important, each person must state clearly what the consequences will be if the young person fails to get help. Parents need to establish and enforce the limits of behavior and state clearly what their continuing expectations of their child are. A lover might break off her relationship; the boss may tell the kids not to come in to work anymore. One important theme participants must emphasize is that they will no longer keep bailing the drug user out of trouble. As one counselor advises, "No more cover-ups. No more clean-ups. No more pick-ups."

Bear in mind, these are not veiled threats, hurled in the heat of emotional stress. They are expressed as logical results of the person's refusal to put his or her life back in order. Everyone involved in the confrontation must be prepared to follow through with these consequences, regardless of the personal pain involved, if they are to wield any power over the substance abuser.

Once these goals have been met, the next step is often to get the person into treatment *immediately.* Many of the interventions in which I've taken part end when the person is brought to our outpatient center for their first day of treatment. In other cases, the addict is handed a suitcase, ushered into a family car, and driven to an inpatient treatment facility. There are other options, but the one chosen by all must be the most likely to succeed.

The strategy of intervention, and the fact that it works so well, is a very big part of the good news about drugs. The reason it works is that, although they often don't realize it, people *do* have power over their loved ones. That power may derive from friendship, from family ties, even from shared life experiences. Sometimes, though, people need a little help to recognize this power and learn how to use it effectively. And each person may think his or her influence may be too small to have much impact on its own.

But organize a group of individuals who care about the user, put them in one room, focus their energies on the drug user's problem—and you have a force that is mighty indeed.

CHAPTER TEN

In Our Schools

There's great news from all across the country. Schools are expanding the "Three *R*s"—reading, writing, and 'rithmetic—and adding a fourth: resisting drugs.

In my view, the goal of education is to help young people deal with the complexities of modern life. No math problem, no spelling problem, is as important as the problem of drug use. By tackling this issue, schools are taking on their rightful share of the responsibility in the fight against drugs.

I'm very excited to hear grade school children describe their school-based prevention programs. In fact, my own daughter was so affected by a DARE program that she was able to apply their teachings about peer pressure to other situations. In this case she was able to stand up to her peers who were urging her to ride a dirt bike in an unsupervised and unsafe situation.

Of course, as we saw in the previous chapter, parents are our first line of defense. Their attitudes, values, and behavior establish a child's fundamental moral framework. But sooner or later parents must send their children out into the real world. Schools help young people make the transition into that world.

Some people think schools shouldn't bother with such issues as drug awareness. They want little Johnny and Judy to keep their minds on "important" topics like the number of degrees in a right angle and whether *I* or *E* comes after *C.* They believe that if you don't talk about things like sex and drugs, they'll just go away.

The good news is that this head-in-the-sand mentality is going the way of the dinosaur. The bad news is it took so much suffering and so many deaths to change some people's minds.

Trouble at School

Eric's father joined a group of parents determined to plumb the depths of the drug problem at the local high school. "One of the other fathers hauled out the school yearbook and demanded that the kids show us who was doing drugs," says Eric's dad. "They told us it would be easier to show who wasn't. My God, there are 2,000 students at that school, and their fast-track, two-income parents don't have any idea what their kids are doing." (From Lamar, Jacob V. "Kids Who Sell Crack." *Time,* May 9, 1988, p. 27.)

In many urban schools, student drug dealers carry mobile phones or wear beepers so they won't miss a customer's call. And get this: In Baltimore, elementary school principals actually had to ban the *fake* beepers that youngsters wear to imitate the drug lords whom they so admire.

At Wesleyan University in Middletown, Connecticut, students staged a two-day drug party. They even promoted the event with posters tacked up around campus. On the first day, billed as the "Smoke Out," they took over a dining hall, smoked pot, and banged on drums and cowbells. On the second day—called "Uncle Duke Day" after the drug-soaked character in the Doonesbury comic strip—they took LSD and played party games. Despite the obvious flouting of the school's antidrug policy, a grand total of one student was arrested. Partygoers saw the university's tolerant attitude as tacit approval of drug use.

Here are some numbers for you to consider:

- Most high school students—78 percent of them, according to PRIDE—have already tried drugs or alcohol.
- A Gallup poll of New Jersey students conducted in late 1989 found that in the previous 30 days, about one student in ten had been asked to sell drugs, and one out of five had been offered drugs.
- Frighteningly, in this same survey, 5 percent of students aged 12 or younger were asked to help sell drugs, and 8 percent of that group said they'd had the opportunity to buy them.
- In another national survey, four out of ten teenagers said drugs were being sold in their schools.
- Nearly one in ten sixth graders said it was "easy" for them to get cocaine and an even higher number felt it was easy to get marijuana.

These clippings from the Fact File prove that children are exposed to illegal drugs during their first years of school, and even earlier, if their parents use drugs at home. And drugs continue to be a threat at every stage of education, from the primary grades through graduate school.

The school-based effort to prevent drug use must begin at the elementary level. To wait until the teenage years is to wait too long.

The Schools Fight Back

Today, many schools share this viewpoint and devote the classroom time necessary to spread the word about drugs. These schools have strong community support—not just money, but other resources as well. As James Wasser, a drug counselor for a New Jersey school district, remarked, "This is the first time that government, education, mental health, police, and communities are involved in a program, and the government has given us enough money to implement it. We've started to unify our services and come together as a whole. That makes me feel good."* Me too.

*Reprinted with permission from the February 1989 issue of *School Security Reports,* Rusting Publications, Port Washington, NY.

Requirements on Drug Prevention Education, Minimum Curriculum Standards, Teacher Certification, and Curriculum Adoption by State *

State	State Requires Substance Abuse Education	Minimum Curriculum Standards Provided	Certification Requirement in Substance Abuse Education for All Teachers	State has Adopted or Designed Prevention Curricula
Alabama	Yes	Yes	No	No
Alaska	No	Yes	No	Yes
Arizona	Yes	Yes	No	No
Arkansas	Yes	Yes	Yes	Yes
California	Yes	Yes	No	No
Colorado	Yes	Yes	No	Yes
Connecticut	Yes	No	No	No
Delaware	Yes	Yes	No	No
D.C.	Yes	Yes	Yes	No
Florida	Yes	Yes	No	No
Georgia	Yes	Yes	No	Yes
Hawaii	No	Yes	No	No
Idaho	Yes	No	No	Yes
Illinois	Yes	Yes	Yes	No
Indiana	Yes	No	Yes	No
Iowa	Yes	Yes	No	No
Kansas	No	No	No	Yes
Kentucky	Yes	Yes	Yes	Yes
Louisiana	Yes	Yes	No	No
Maine	Yes	Yes	No	No
Maryland	Yes	Yes	No	Yes
Massachusetts	Yes	No	No	Yes
Michigan	No	Yes	No	Yes
Minnesota	Yes	Yes	Yes	No
Mississippi	No	No	No	No
Missouri	No	No	Yes	No
Montana	No	No	No	No
Nebraska	Yes	No	No	Yes
Nevada	Yes	Yes	Yes	No
New Hampshire	Yes	No	No	Yes
New Jersey	Yes	No	Yes	No
New Mexico	Yes	Yes	No	No
New York	Yes	Yes	Yes	Yes
North Carolina	No	No	No	No
North Dakota	Yes	No	No	No
Ohio	Yes	No	Yes	No
Oklahoma	No	No	No	No

continued

State	State Requires Substance Abuse Education	Minimum Curriculum Standards Provided	Certification Requirement in Substance Abuse Education for All Teachers	State has Adopted or Designed Prevention Curricula
Oregon	Yes	No	No	No
Pennsylvania	Yes	Yes	No	Yes
Rhode Island	Yes	Yes	No	No
South Carolina	Yes	No	No	No
South Dakota	No	No	No	No
Tennessee	No	Yes	No	No
Texas	Yes	Yes	No	Yes
Utah	Yes	Yes	No	Yes
Vermont	Yes	Yes	No	No
Virginia	Yes	Yes	No	Yes
Washington	Yes	Yes	No	No
West Virginia	Yes	Yes	No	No
Wisconsin	Yes	Yes	No	No
Wyoming	No	No	No	No
Total with requirement	**39**	**32**	**11**	**17**

* *Source:* ***Report to Congress and the White House on the Nature and Effectiveness of Federal, State, and Local Drug Prevention Education Programs.*** *Washington, D.C.: U.S. Departments of Education and Health and Human Services, October 1987.*

What does it take for a school to develop and implement an antidrug program? So many schools have done it successfully that others can profit from their experience. Let me describe the overall goals and strategies that any such program should have.

Policy The battle begins with a firm commitment: Tobacco, alcohol, and illicit drugs have no place in the learning environment and the school will not tolerate their use. The school must put this policy in writing. It must then communicate the policy clearly to everyone in the school, enforce it fairly and consistently, and *reinforce* it by teaching prevention. As one school district superintendent stated, "Policy must be the school's number one priority, or else nothing else flows. Policy must be strong and backed up all along the chain, from the district office to the classroom."

The elements of good policy are simple and require little more than common sense. Basically, the policy needs to define clearly, and in ways consistent with state laws, exactly what drugs and forms of drug use are covered. Prescription medications, for example, would not be covered, but alcohol should be. The policy must also spell out when and where drugs are prohibited: on school grounds, at school-sponsored functions, and so on. There must be a list of consequences violators can expect. Lastly, the policy must describe the process by which students will be sent for treatment and how they may be reinstated in school. Such procedures must be handled confidentially and with due regard for the student's civil rights.

Three fourths of the country's 16,490 school districts have now developed such policies. Of these, over 90 percent require that kids using drugs be suspended or receive counseling, and that the parents, the police, or both be notified of the problem. (See Chart on pages 190–91.)

In support of the movement, the U.S. Department of Education has created guidelines to insure that school substance abuse programs will work. After the basic antidrug policy is in place, these guidelines call on schools to:

- Develop and enforce standards for all school personnel concerning their professional conduct and their roles in teaching drug prevention.
- Find out how severe the drug problem is in their area through surveys and consultations with law enforcement officials and parents, and inform the community of the results.
- Select a comprehensive drug prevention curriculum and implement the program at every level from kindergarten through twelfth grade.
- Involve parents and other community leaders in the program.
- Refer students with drug problems for counseling and treatment, and arrange for special education as needed.
- Include the antidrug message in school activities and events, and encourage this practice in family and community activities.

• Create written guidelines stating how schools and law enforcement agencies can cooperate in presenting antidrug programs and spelling out procedures for intervening on school grounds.

• Evaluate the program regularly and make changes as needed.

Personnel Policy is useless without people. For antidrug programs to work, everyone—from superintendent to student—must play a role.

The superintendent is a vital element, the person who provides leadership, coordinates resources in the district and the community, and supports others as they work toward their goals.

The principal develops the resources within an individual school and acts as a liaison between students, parents, and the district. The principal sets the tone for antidrug education and sees that its message gets across.

Administrators are the top brass in the school drug war, but *teachers* are the troops battling it out on the front lines. They need good training to handle the explosive situations they may encounter, and they need ammunition in the form of hard facts, training in problem-solving skills, and access to good teaching materials.

Another player on the team is the *substance awareness coordinator.* Having a specialist on staff, one who is dedicated to the drug issue, is an invaluable source of information and guidance. It also sends a clear signal to the student body about the seriousness with which the school regards the problem.

Some of you may ask, "In these days of tight budgets, can we really afford to have an extra person on the payroll?" I answer with another question: "Can we afford not to?"

Look at the impact such a person can have. In Newark, where the school district hired a number of substance-awareness coordinators, drug use declined swiftly and significantly. "Just Say No" clubs were formed in 25 Newark schools, with more on the way. The coordinators developed a touring puppet program to spark discussions about drugs among chil-

What Students Can Do

- Learn the effects and risks of drugs.
- Study the symptoms of drug use.
- Be aware of the organizations and people available to help when friends or family members are in trouble.
- Recognize peer pressure and learn how to resist it.
- Know the school's rules on drugs and how to make the policy work.
- Find out the school's procedures for reporting drug offenses.
- Understand what the community antidrug laws and penalties are.
- Realize that these laws were designed to protect individuals —users and nonusers alike—and society.
- Express opposition to drugs whenever the opportunity arises.
- Participate in school and community discussions about the drug problem.
- Set a positive example.
- Teach other students, especially younger ones, about the harmful effects of drugs.
- Talk with parents and encourage them to join the fight.
- Join or start an antidrug club or drug-free activity.
- Encourage drug-using friends to get help.

(Adapted from U.S. Department of Education. *Schools Without Drugs: What Works,* 1989, pp. 33–35.)

dren from kindergarten through fourth grade. Students have even created a performing arts group where they write, produce, and star in their own antidrug musical plays. If anyone can think of a more positive, upbeat, or effective way to get the message across to kids, I'd love to hear about it.

Students themselves must be considered members of the team. Remember, peer pressure works two ways: It can cause kids to succumb to temptation, but it can also give them the strength to resist it. The best antidrug programs shore up students' resistance and empower them to help their peers avoid

One Peer Counseling Program

Responsibility Pledge for a Peer Counselor
R. H. Watkins High School
Jones County, Mississippi

As a drug education peer counselor you have the opportunity to help the youth of our community develop to their full potential without the interference of illegal drug use. It is a responsibility you must not take lightly. Therefore, please read the following responsibilities you will be expected to fulfill next school year and discuss them with your parents or guardians.

Responsibilities of a Peer Counselor

- Understand and be able to clearly state your beliefs and attitudes about drug use among teens and adults.
- Remain drug free.
- Maintain an average of C or better in all classes.
- Maintain a citizenship average of B or better.
- Participate in some club or extracurricular activity that emphasizes the positive side of school life.
- Successfully complete training for the program, including, for example, units on the identification and symptoms of drug abuse, history and reasons for drug abuse, and the legal/economic aspects of drug abuse.
- Successfully present monthly programs on drug abuse in each of the elementary and junior high schools of the school system, and to community groups, churches, and statewide groups as needed.
- Participate in rap sessions or individual counseling sessions with school students.
- Attend at least one Jones County Drug Council meeting per year, attend the annual Drug Council Awards Banquet, work in the Drug Council Fair exhibit and in any Drug Council workshops, if needed.
- Grades and credit for Drug Education will be awarded on successful completion of and participation in all the above-stated activities.

(Signed by the student and the parents or guardians.)

(Reprinted with permission from O. David Jones, Drug Education Coordinator, Laurel School District, Laurel, MS.)

the dangers of drugs. A timely word from a concerned friend can make all the difference. Students can also help if they are shown how to report drug use without putting themselves or others at risk. (See Box on page 194.)

Some antidrug programs suggest peer counseling, in which teenaged volunteers are trained to advise their fellow students. Peer counseling is controversial. There is concern that without careful monitoring, a student counselor may say exactly the wrong thing at exactly the wrong time. It is best, say some experts, to leave such matters to professionals. On the other hand, many schools with peer counseling programs report good results.

I believe that few things have as much impact on young people in trouble as having friends of their own age and background express concern and offer a helping hand. I think the objections to peer counseling can be met by providing good training and supervision. For an example of how one school in Mississippi designed a peer counseling program, see the Box on page 195.

Other resources that schools should not overlook are the *student-run media*—newspapers, literary magazines, drama clubs, even closed-circuit television or radio productions. The school officials in charge of antidrug education should work with the students and the faculty advisers in charge of these media, first to encourage them to cover drug issues on a regular basis, and second to make sure their information is complete and accurate. Properly used, student-to-student communication can contribute much to the campus atmosphere of zero tolerance.

Another option to consider: There are workshops available in which kids meet with trained representatives to develop and present an antidrug program. As an example, PRIDE promotes a series of events it calls "America's Pride" aimed at students at the middle school and high school level. After a day of intensive rap sessions and rehearsal, participants stage a revue complete with skits, songs, and dances. The antidrug message comes through loud and clear; one reporter described the event as a "cram course in love."

How Schools Can Involve Parents

- Talk about antidrug programs at meetings of the parent-teacher organization and at school open houses.
- Publicize antidrug programs and activities.
- Include drug prevention as part of the orientation program for new students and their parents.
- Sponsor a seminar for parents on the facts about drug abuse.
- Involve parents in planning and implementing antidrug programs.
- Draw on parents' skills to make presentations to students—for example, ask parents who are nurses, pharmacists, or law enforcement officials to speak.
- Invite parents to assist in school activities such as alcohol-free proms and graduation parties.
- Require parents and students to attend a driver's education session about the hazards of driving under the influence of drugs or alcohol.

(Adapted from U.S. Department of Education. *Schools Without Drugs: The Challenge,* March/April 1989, p. 10.)

Parents Parents are a child's first and most important teachers. They must be recruited to participate in any school antidrug program if it is to succeed (see Box above). As Sue Schaumburg, a volunteer who chairs the drug education committee in her son's school in suburban Kansas City, observes, "Without support from parents, kids in a 'Just Say No' program are like a ship without an anchor, a rudder, a working radio, or a harbor to come home to. The kids just drift along. They have nothing to steer them on the right course. They pick up conflicting signals. And they have no place where they feel snug and secure."

It helps to open and maintain contact between parents and teachers through regular meetings. In such sessions, a child's problems at home or at school, such as absenteeism, may crop up and get talked about. Another strategy is to make sure each parent receives, reads, and signs a copy of the school's antidrug policy. School officials should work with parents to provide extra help for students who are having trouble and to organize after-school activities that prevent a child from having to go home to an empty house.

Schools can offer workshops to train parents on preventing drug use. (PRIDE, for example, offers the "Parent to Parent" seminars, and there are others available). Having parents go along on field trips, assist in sports programs, and chaperone parties at school or in their homes can make a huge difference. It also helps to hire an active, concerned parent to serve as a full-time liaison between the school and other parents. Another option is to assign homework that calls for direct parental involvement, such as having the student "interview" parents about their drug attitudes.

Sometimes bringing parents into the program takes a little ingenuity. In many families both parents work. All parents, but especially single parents, have enormous demands on their time. It may not be realistic to expect them to attend parent-teacher conferences during after-school hours. One solution is for schools to reach out to employers and urge them to grant their employees time off to become involved in school antidrug programs.

Designing the Curriculum

Part of the good news about drugs is that educators today have many options in choosing an antidrug program that's right for their schools. The booklet "Drug Prevention Curricula: A Guide to Selection and Implementation," published by U.S. Department of Education, is a splendid overview of what everyone concerned in this vital decision should know. I can only touch on some of the main issues in this chapter; for other sources of information, see the Appendix.

Finding the Program The first decision is whether to buy an existing program, complete with workbooks, video instruction modules, on-site training by visiting consultants—the works. Such programs can cost thousands of dollars for a single set of materials and training. Or schools may choose to adapt such a program and tailor it to their own needs. Many schools on tight budgets go this route. Another option is to develop their own curriculum from the ground up. One method of doing so is to work with local law enforcement agencies, thus spreading the cost among the interested parties. Often the laws of an individual state determine the choice. In California, for example, schools must use programs that have a specific content and set of procedures. Half of the states have bought commercial packages or use ones developed by the state itself.

Schools must make sure the program includes adequate training; likewise, administrators must support the program by making sure enough classroom time—and money—is available. Also, schools must work hard to reach those students who most need this information: the high-risk students, the truants, and those with learning disabilities. Conversely, gifted students may be bored or uninterested if the program is too simpleminded; their needs must be addressed as well.

Be aware that so far there is no national consensus on exactly which curricula work best. Schools should research the matter carefully before making their decision, just as consumers do their homework before buying a new car or refrigerator.

Goals No matter what structure or materials they use, all antidrug programs must have the same goals: To teach the value of healthy minds and bodies, and to point out how drugs destroy them; to teach understanding and respect for the law; to train students to recognize and resist pressure to use drugs; and to promote drug-free activities.

Some warnings: If a drug program takes a passive approach —presenting the bare facts without taking a firm antidrug stand —pass it by. Information without judgment does nothing to curb students' appetite for drugs; it just piques their curiosity. Give them the facts, sure, but spell it out loud and clear: *Drug use in any form is unacceptable.*

Also, some antidrug programs say teachers should promote open discussion by revealing their own past indiscretions. *Wrong!* Teachers must maintain the distinction between themselves and their students, between adult and adolescent. Equally wrong is the notion that students should discuss or confess their own drug experiences. Doing so may only increase curiosity among students who don't use drugs. It may also confuse the issues, forcing kids to take sides against each other or make harsh judgments.

Content In shopping for a curriculum, schools should read the materials carefully to make sure the program takes an active stand against drugs based on solid facts. The message must echo at every level, from kindergarten through senior year.

The content must be geared to the appropriate age group. In kindergarten through third grade, the emphasis should be on the wonder of the human body and the brain, and on the importance of keeping them healthy—physically, psychologically, and socially. Kids this age are capable of seeing the difference between a medicine and a drug. One teacher in Brooklyn makes this point to her five-year-olds by showing them cartoon drawings that carry a simple message: "Only sick people should be taking drugs." By the end of this stage, kids should know about specific illicit drugs and how they are different from the ones a doctor gives them. They should know that people can become sick on drugs but that there are ways to help those people. They can do science lessons that teach them about hazardous materials, or reading lessons that emphasize warning signs and danger signals. Even at this tender age, they can begin to grasp the concept of law and what it means to do something outside the law.

The emphasis in grades four through six changes. Kids should know how to identify specific drugs and understand why they are dangerous, especially for growing bodies. At this stage they can understand addiction and how pressure from peers or from the media promotes drug use. Because they have more freedom to move about, these kids need to know how to stay out of trouble on the streets and playgrounds. They should realize that breaking laws leads to consequences. They also should learn how to get help for themselves or anyone who has a substance abuse problem.

In middle schools kids reach puberty; they begin to date; access to drugs is easier; peer pressure increases; and chronic mistrust of adults sets in. Drug programs must recognize and address these dramatic changes in kids' lives. Students need to learn the effects of drugs on the brain, heart, lungs, muscles, and reproductive organs. They must understand chemical dependency and how it affects society. English classes can assign novels that portray the horrors of drugs; social studies classes can trace the impact of the drug epidemic, including the spread of AIDS; science and biology classes can explore the actions of chemicals on the body, while physical education classes can hammer home the point that drugs—including steroids—don't improve performance, they destroy it.

In high school, students begin to transform into adult citizens. They must learn about the legal, social, and economic impact of drug use—not just on themselves but on others. The basic theme should be that use of drugs can destroy their lives now and for years to come—by keeping them out of college, preventing them from getting the job they want, by saddling them with a police record. Boys as well as girls should know the effects of drugs on a baby in the womb.

To my way of thinking, the buck doesn't stop in high school. We need to keep sounding the alarm all the way through college and graduate schools. Sadly, many students in medical schools—*medical schools!*—are less disapproving of drug use than their twelfth-grade counterparts. Even though they have access to the entire body of scientific literature, over 30 percent of medical school students rely on close friends or television as their source of knowledge about cocaine. I urge that medical schools include a course on drugs as a requirement for every first-year student. I'll even go a step further: They should require a urine test—with clean results—before considering a candidate for admission. We doctors must put our own house in order if we expect to end drug use among our patients.

Resistance Skills The best antidrug programs teach modern-day survival skills along with the facts. The programs develop the personal traits that help people resist drugs: high self-esteem, sound judgment, ability to handle stress, strength to resist peer pressure, and mental agility to resolve the conflicting messages about drugs emanating from home and society. Kids can learn to use these skills just as they learn martial arts —as a form of self-defense. Teachers need to point out that, sure, we all feel hopeless and depressed at times, but there are other solutions beside drugs.

It's true that many people use drugs in part to compensate for their lack of a positive self-image. But just building up a sense of personal worth isn't enough. The successful program will help boost kids' sense of themselves, and make clear the link between low self-esteem and drug use.

Another key skill is resistance. Among the proven methods of resistance are the Cold Shoulder (ignoring entreaties to use drugs), the Broken Record (constantly repeating refusals— "No! No! No!"), the Good Excuse ("My mom would kill me!"), and Strength in Numbers (hanging out with non-drug users).

Joseph Berger, writing in *The New York Times,* reports that schools in Kansas City, Kansas, give students 15 lessons a year in resisting drugs. One technique has students improvise scenes addressing various issues. In one such exercise Monica called Danita a "wimp" for turning down marijuana. Danita in turn used the ploy known as "reverse pressure"—she simply snapped back that she would tell all their friends that Monica's momma "still tucks you in at night."

Do these methods work? In one survey, 13 percent of students who *didn't* take the class smoked cigarettes, 9 percent drank booze, and 7 percent used pot. But among those who *did* take the class, only 3 percent used tobacco, 4 percent alcohol, and 3 percent marijuana. I'm convinced.

It may be harder to reach some people, such as older students or those who live in the inner city. These kids may think there's no way for them to escape their background except through drugs. Because they have nothing to lose, trying to simply scare them away from drugs simply won't work. An antidrug program must recognize this problem and address it specifically if it is to work in an urban setting.

Time How much time should be devoted to antidrug training? In New York, the law requires that students receive at least eight hours a year. However, some drug enforcement officials feel that even 25 hours a year isn't enough. And of course, quality is better than quantity. It's a waste of time to give a hundred-hour course taught by ill-informed or ineffective teachers, or one that doesn't start until high school or that is presented by outsiders who don't know how to communicate with students.

Assessing Results It's also important to measure results through grading or some other means. Without this assessment —a kind of Nielsen ratings for drug programs—there is no way to know if the message is getting across. Schools can use such data as police records of drug-related incidents, statistics on the use of treatment and referral services, student surveys, feedback from staff, parents, and the community, student participation in drug-free activities, and so on. Equally important, schools need to study this feedback to learn whether the program should be improved—or dumped altogether.

Antidrug Programs in Action

I could fill the rest of this book with exciting stories of how specific schools have confronted the drug problem and conquered it. I'll have to be content, however, with just a few outstanding examples.

Project TRUST: This program in Dade County, Florida, focuses on community awareness of drug abuse, counseling for students and parents, and referrals for treatment. Among other measures, students are forbidden from wearing clothing that promotes alcohol or drug use. Though this is just a small symbolic step, it makes sense to me. Within a year the number of students disciplined for drug offenses fell from 100 to 25; a survey of eighth graders showed a 35 percent drop in drug use from the year before.

Project HOPE: Developed in Central Valley, California, the name stands for Helping Other People Everywhere. Here the emphasis is on crime prevention, forming a student support network, and developing a library of information about drugs. Through this program, students set up Neighborhood Watch Programs; police report a significant drop in vandalism in the community.

Project SCOPE: The name refers to the South Carolina Coping Skills Project. This program, aimed at kids at high risk, focuses on learning proper behavior and assertiveness, managing anxiety, making decisions, and developing communication and social skills. Parents are shown how to help students apply these lessons in the home. There has been a big drop in alcohol use among those who participated in the program.

Growing Healthy: This program, developed in part by the New York Academy of Medicine, is being used in over 40 states. Aimed at kids in kindergarten through seventh grade, it emphasizes nutrition and hygiene. In one exercise, kids blow into straws to inflate a calf's lung with air. The point is then dramatized that smoking tobacco or marijuana can destroy the lungs' ability to pump oxygen.

Project Graduation: This is an effort by the National Highway Transportation Safety Administration that helps schools sponsor drug-and-alcohol-free graduation parties.

Be Smart! Stay Smart! Don't Start: The Office for Substance Abuse Prevention, part of the Department of Health and Human Services, launched this program in 1987. Aimed at kids aged eight through 12, the program creates videos and public service announcements and sponsors antidrug activities that focus on the concept of gateway drugs. Program materials are available through RADAR—the Regional Alcohol and Drug Awareness Resource, with offices in every state.

SPECDA: This New York City program, whose name means the School Program to Educate and Control Drug Abuse, was developed in conjunction with law enforcement personnel. SPECDA stresses peer counseling, drug-free clubs, self-help groups, car washes, variety shows, dances, puppet shows, and rap sessions.

Here's Looking at You 2000: According to the substance abuse coordinator for schools in Teaneck, New Jersey, this comprehensive kindergarten-through-12th-grade program has emerged as the "elite" curriculum in the United States. During one of the 30 lessons in this program, given in a Kansas City school, second graders pretended they were organs of the body: lungs pumping, hearts beating. The instructor then asked them to imagine what would happen if they put drugs into those organs, and if they just kept putting in more and more drugs. By the end of the exercise, the children ran around the room and flailed their arms until they were exhausted. The point was driven home: Eventually, drugs will wear you down.

Project STAR: This 15-lesson program was developed by the Ewing Marion Kauffmann Foundation, a charitable organization started by the owner of the Kansas City Royals in the aftermath of publicity about cocaine use by members of the team. As we saw earlier, Project STAR teaches kids like Monica and Danita how to build up their skills at resisting pressure to try drugs.

Project DARE: Founded and headquartered in Los Angeles, Project DARE is a cooperative effort between law enforcement and local schools. In this program, police officers enter the classroom to provide factual information on drug abuse. I have personally enjoyed working with this project.

I could go on, but you see my point. Our schools—more precisely, our administrators, teachers, parents, students, and government agencies—have confronted the challenge of drug abuse and have devised solutions that are creative, effective—and life saving.

I'd say that earns an A +.

CHAPTER ELEVEN

In Our Workplaces

Illicit drugs are used in all occupations and professions, from large factories to small businesses, from the boardroom to the toolroom.
—*The White House Conference for a Drug-Free America, Final Report, June 1988*

In 1984, I predicted that drug abuse in the workplace and the drug testing of employees would soon become major issues in America. At that time my prediction was usually met with either blank stares or skeptical comments like "Aren't you exaggerating the problem?" Or, "Why would a company worry about what its workers did on the weekend?" The implicit rationale behind this skepticism was that somehow drug abusers could turn off the effects of their drug use—that a joint smoked at lunchtime would make a airplane mechanic incapable of completing a simple sentence but not interfere with his ability to repair a jet engine. Or that a weekend-long, cocaine-fueled party would somehow not hinder an accountant from balancing the books on Monday morning. At that time there was a prevailing attitude in America that drug use should be tolerated.

But in 1984 my office began to be deluged with calls from corporations asking for help in confronting an ever-growing problem: employee drug abuse. High-level executive and mid-level managers alike would pepper me with some very basic questions: "How do I tell if my employees have a drug problem?"; "Why is my evening shift doing so poorly?"; "Why is the turnover rate so high on my assembly line?" Business in general has always had a drug problem, one that they either didn't know about or chose to ignore. But in the early 1980s, with the increase in cocaine and marijuana use, business began to see just how devastating employee drug abuse could be. Finally, business realized that its single greatest resource was being slowly devoured by drugs and the tolerant atmosphere that allowed drug use to thrive. It was that resource, namely our workforce, that has made it possible for us to create and enjoy a standard of living unparalleled in the world. Our economic growth, as well as large measures of the social progress we enjoy as a nation, are due to the efforts of efficient and dedicated workers.

Drugs and alcohol threaten that progress. They destroy productivity, reducing the quality of goods and services and increasing their cost. Drug use adds to the already enormous burden of health care through absenteeism, accidents, and the need for treatment. It causes enormous suffering, disrupts lives, ruins careers, and demolishes whole companies.

Drug use costs society as much as *$60 to $100 billion a year.* Worst of all, drugs cost lives. Medical bills are just part of the picture. Other costs include crime, law enforcement expenses, and lowered real estate values. As Robert B. Reich, a political economist, told *The New York Times,* "Narcotics is one of America's major industries, right up there with consumer electronics, automobiles, and steelmaking. . . . In fact, it is like a reverse industry, tearing things down rather than producing anything." (Copyright 1989 by *The New York Times.* Reprinted by permission.)

The good news: Business is fighting back. Companies now see drugs as the biggest threat to their future. A survey in late 1989 found that 64 percent of managers believe substance abuse is the nation's most critical labor and employment problem. Just a year before, AIDS had topped the list. But more than just *seeing* the problem, businesses—working jointly with their employees and their unions—are *doing* something about it.

- As part of their benefits package, companies offer employee assistance programs to help workers and their families with drug problems.

• In their job advertisements, businesses announce prominently that their workplace is drug-free—and that any applicants had better be, too.

• Acknowledging their role in solving society's problems, companies contribute their energy and resources to antidrug education through public conferences, media articles, broadcasts, advertisements, and other creative strategies.

Companies—even in the recession of 1991—know it's in their own best interests to take a stand against drugs. When it comes to employees, it costs a lot less to rehabilitate than terminate. As a spokesman for a major car manufacturer observed, his company's drug policy is not designed to find substance abusers and kick them out; instead, "our major objective is to turn them back into the successes they once were." And Peter Besinger, one of this country's experts on drug abuse in the workplace, has pointed out it is more cost-effective for a company to treat an employee with a drug problem than to go through the expense of hiring and training a new employee. And as Richard Lesher, president of the United States Chamber of Commerce, told *The New York Times:* "Employers have the most effective weapon in the war on drugs: the paycheck."

Scope of the Problem

There's no doubt that drug use by workers, left unchallenged, threatens to undermine our economy. An estimated 20 million jobs in this country are now held by people who use marijuana, amphetamines, or cocaine. A few years ago, in the first round of government-ordered drug tests, significant drug use was found among members of the Secret Service, air traffic controllers, nuclear and chemical weapons security personnel, and aviation safety employees.

A survey conducted through the 800-COCAINE helpline found that three out of four people currently using cocaine had gone to work under the influence of drugs. Of that group, more than 20 percent said they did so frequently. Thirty-eight percent said they bought their drugs from one of their coworkers —and nearly one out of thee made purchases *on the company premises.*

No wonder Bob Frederick, manager of health-service programs for Xerox, was moved to remark: "If you want to tear a country apart, you don't have to use bombs. Just make drugs available, and it will self-destruct."

Want more numbers? I got 'em for you.

- As many as 65 percent of the young people entering the workforce have used illegal drugs.
- The National Institute on Drug Abuse (NIDA) estimates that one out of eight workers between the ages of 26 and 35 abuse drugs, including alcohol, while at work.
- For younger workers aged 18 and 25, the numbers (and the people!) are even higher: 20 percent use drugs on the job.
- Drug users incur medical costs that on average are *three times as high* as the rest of a company's employees.
- Drug users are absent from work twice as often as non-using employees.
- Users are five times as likely to be involved in accidents when off the job.

Workers on Drugs

Numbers are fine, but alone they don't give a true picture of human suffering. Let me show you how drug use in the workplace affects people by telling you of some patients we have treated.

Typical of the problem is Luke, a 34-year-old manager for a large East Coast banking firm. Luke reported that every morning, before he had even turned on the shower, he snorted a couple of lines of coke to "jump-start my motor." Before leaving for work, he would toss back a couple of hits of vodka in lieu of breakfast to quell his anxiety.

By the time he arrived at the office his early-morning buzz had worn off, so Luke would do another couple of lines, often with a coworker, a personnel director from whom he often bought his supply. There or four times a day they would signal each other over the telephone intercom system—the code words were "It's tea time"—and head for the washroom to toot up.

In time Luke began borrowing money from the company to support his habit; when those funds dried up, he simply shifted to stealing through what he called "creative accounting."

Luke's undoing came during a crucial late-afternoon planning session. He had been on a coke-induced emotional roller coaster the entire day, and was already tired, irritable, and a little paranoid. Twice within 45 minutes he left to visit the men's room, muttering something about "too much coffee." Normally Luke presented his ideas with clarity and enthusiasm, but today his thoughts were rambling and unfocused. His judgment had become cloudy; his energy level had obviously plummeted.

His boss eyed Luke's performance—not to mention his dripping nose—with suspicion. Later, he asked Luke to talk with one of the company's in-house counselors. When Luke denied that there was anything wrong—"I'm just coming down with a cold"—the boss upgraded the suggestion to a demand. After seeing the counselor, Luke was referred to Fair Oaks for evaluation and possible treatment.

Luke's belief—his illusion, really—that the drug helped him in his work set the trap for continued and escalating use. He had thought cocaine boosted his creativity, gave him the stamina to put in 50- and 60-hour weeks, and helped him earn, as he put it, "more money than I'd thought I'd see in my entire life." Eventually, though, he hit a brick wall: The drug he took to boost his performance turned on him, and ruined him instead.

After treatment, Luke was able to pick up the pieces of his life. He realized how self-destructive he had been. He found ways to make up for the damage he had done—not just to himself, but to his employers and his family. Today he volunteers as a drug counselor at an outpatient clinic.

Luke's story highlights two important points. First, professionals or high-level employees are not immune to addiction, and in many cases they must be threatened with the loss of their job before they get treatment. Second, knowing there is a job waiting for them can make a big difference in their motivation to get better.

Some companies and those who run them are still blind to drug use in the workplace. Often supervisors or peers are aware of the problem but they ignore it or cover it up. Sometimes this happens because the company has no written guidelines for dealing with substance abuse, and so they must make up their policy as they go along. That approach just won't cut it.

Drugs on the Job

Why do people use drugs on the job? There are many reasons. As we saw in Luke's story, he believed drugs would *enhance performance.*

Contrast that with Hollis, who worked in a steel mill. Every day Hollis would take his position at the start of the shift and think to himself, "Oh boy—another ten hours of shoveling metal chips into a bucket." He used marijuana, he said, so that "at least his mind would be broadcasting in color even though his life was black and white." For Hollis, drug use was driven by *boredom.*

The *"burnout" syndrome* may also contribute to the problem. Burnout can happen to anyone, from athletes to art museum directors, if they begin to feel that the conflicts between their aspirations and their limits, or the pressures of their jobs, become overwhelming. Some people feel drugs will help them manage these stresses.

Often drug use is fueled simply by *availability of drugs* or by an *attitude of tolerance by employers.* Jaqui, an aspiring actress and a hostess at a popular New York restaurant, said she started using cocaine because everyone else who worked there did. After the restaurant closed, the whole staff, including the owner, often went to someone's apartment or to an "after-hours" club where they snorted themselves into oblivion. "I felt that if I didn't use drugs the others might treat me like an outsider and I wouldn't be assigned to any shifts," Jaqui reported.

Which drugs do people use at work? You can essentially divide illicit drugs into two groups: the ones people use at work and those they don't. Cocaine, alcohol, and marijuana are the top three abused substances in the workplace. These drugs are popular because they can be integrated readily into work activities. Because such drugs as LSD, heroin, and "angel dust" cause agitation, hallucinations, drowsiness, or other strange behavior, they are seldom used on the job since they are too easy to detect. A person who drinks his lunch and still manages to toddle through the rest of the day is a much less conspicuous substance abuser than a heroin addict who falls asleep at her desk.

Our experience with patients confirms that it's hard to spot a worker's problem with marijuana early. Abuse becomes apparent only after a prolonged period of time (or with drug testing). Even after prolonged use it may take some calamity—a tumble from a ladder or an attempt to relocate a telephone pole using the fender of one's car—before the problem becomes obvious. But for chronic marijuana abusers who have only marginal skills or who have psychological problems, it's just a matter of time before their inability to do their job, their negative attitudes, their poor memory, and their lax work habits lead to an accident, demotion, or their dismissal (unless they are saddled with a job that is far below their potential).

It's ironic, but patients are often less ashamed to admit they have a problem if their substance of abuse is cocaine rather than some other drug. For some people, cocaine powder is still seen as a sign of affluence, of being a "high roller"; alcoholism, by contrast, is stigmatized as a problem of weakness and loss of control. As Luke told me, "There's no reason *not* to use coke at work. It's easy to carry, it doesn't take long to dose yourself, and usually no one has any idea that you've done it."

Since the advent of crack, smokable cocaine has become

the drug of choice—especially among the young. While crack may not bring the user the same aura of wealth and social class as cocaine powder, it does have a "happening" association. And many substance abuse counselors report growing numbers of people who use two or more drugs in combination. It's getting harder to keep pace with these multiple addictions, which, counselors say, are the biggest killer.

What's the harm in using drugs at work? An 800-COCAINE survey in May of 1988 assessed the impact of drugs on work. Forty-five percent of the women calling and 61 percent of the men stated that their drug use had caused them to miss time at work, through absences, lateness, or having to leave early. Asked if they had ever lost a job because of drugs, 18 percent of the men and 13 percent of the women said yes.

Interestingly, a lot of the 800-COCAINE calls we received when we started the hotline came in on Sunday nights. Callers often told us that they had a meeting with the boss in the morning and they were scared. As one caller said, "I'm either going to get a raise and a promotion or I'm going to get fired. The weird thing is, I don't have any idea which it'll be." That's another side effect of drugs: Loss of touch with reality.

Many accidents on the job can be attributed to drug use. From 1975 to 1985, for example, use of drugs and alcohol caused at least 48 train wrecks, resulting in 37 deaths, 80 injuries, and $34 million in property damage. In the years since that study, the problem has grown worse; in one 1987 accident, an Amtrak passenger train carrying drug-impaired crew members collided with a Conrail freight train near Baltimore, killing 16 people and injuring 175. Untold numbers of airplane wrecks, car crashes, and other less violent accidents can also be traced more or less directly to drugs.

Even if the employee does not actually use drugs or alcohol while at work, there can be residual problems: hangovers, poor judgment, irritability, sudden mood swings, drowsiness, preoccupation with attaining the drug, personality changes, and a general inability to function. Many users vow never to use drugs at work, but at lunch or at five o'clock they make a beeline for their drugs. They think about drugs on the job, use company time (not to mention company telephones, company premises, and, frequently, company money) to set up a drug buy, and most likely buy or sell drugs to coworkers. Employees whose drug use causes trouble with wives and families often can't leave those problems behind when they step into the office in the morning.

What Companies Can Do

No matter what business it is involved in, no matter what its size, any company can and must take steps to prevent drug use by its workers. The first step is to make the fight against drugs a priority. For managers to dismiss substance abuse in the workplace as a "cost of doing business" is wrong. A department store wouldn't tolerate stealing by its employees. By the same token, no business should tolerate the loss of time, energy, and quality caused by drug abuse.

Company Policy Companies must establish strong antidrug policies that cover every employee, from the CEO to the mailroom clerk. As in the schools, that policy must be put in writing and distributed to everyone. *Policy must be based on the principle that we are fighting drugs—not the people using them.*

To be effective, any policy must give people the power to act. Managers and supervisors must have the resources, the authority, and the courage to confront their coworkers in trouble. They must know how to steer their employees toward the help they need. And they must show compassion and fairness as they support their fellow workers in their struggle.

By 1989, 13 percent of all businesses, employing 43 percent of all workers except those who work on farms, had set up formal written policies against drug use. Of companies with 5,000 or more employees, 83 percent had such policies, as did 6 percent of businesses with fewer than 10 employees. The good news is that so many companies have taken this crucial

Company Antidrug Policy Statement

1. Almost any human problem—physical illness, mental or emotional illness, finances, marital or family distress, alcoholism, drug abuse, legal problems—can be successfully treated if it is identified in its early stages and if the person is given appropriate care.
2. The purpose of this policy is to assure employees of the XYZ Company that assistance is available to help resolve such problems in an effective and confidential manner.
3. Problems causing unsatisfactory job performance will be handled in keeping with the company's procedures governing health and personnel. All records will be kept in strictest confidence.
4. When necessary, a leave of absence may be granted for treatment or rehabilitation for alcoholism and/or drug abuse.
5. Employees are encouraged to voluntarily seek confidential counseling and information.
6. Employees in the program will be encouraged to secure adequate medical, rehabilitative, counseling, or other services, as needed.
7. It will be the responsibility of the employee to comply with the referrals to assess the problem, and to follow the recommendations of the caregiver.
8. The referral source is available to the families of our employees as well.

(Adapted with permission of Carolina Division Bowater Incorporated. From U.S. Department of Labor *What Works: Workplaces Without Drugs.*)

step. Eventually, though, *all* businesses must do so if we are to win our war on drugs.

For an example of antidrug policy, based on one developed by the Bowater Carolina Company, see the Box above.

In order to work, a policy must address the issue of how to spot an employee with a substance abuse problem. One measure is to track the usual signs of trouble: accidents, theft, security breaches, absenteeism, and worker compensation claims. Studies show that about 50 percent of such incidents are related to drug or alcohol abuse. Another way is to meet with representatives of different divisions, including occupational health and safety, personnel, security, and unions, to discuss and define the problem. It also helps to ask workers for their views.

A good policy is one that makes the family aware of the company's antidrug stance and its program for helping its workers. Often, it's the spouse of the employee who first raises the alarm. Typically, for example, a wife may call the company's medical director and say something like "Either my spouse is having an affair or he's a drug addict. He's uninterested in sex, or me, he ignores his children, and we're just falling apart." Such a comment can set the wheels in motion and salvage an employee.

The Employee Assistance Program (EAP) A policy gives a company's antidrug effort its backbone; the EAP gives it flesh and blood. These lifesaving programs work because they take into account the needs of individuals as well as the companies they work for. At this point, nearly 30 million workers are employed in businesses that provide EAPs—three times as many as in 1985, when crack cocaine first burst on the scene. Among the organizations whose EAPs are considered models of success are the Association of Flight Attendants; AT&T; General Motors and the United Auto Workers; IBM; Xerox; and even the St. Louis Symphony.

The modern-day concept of an EAP evolved from programs developed during the 1940s that focused on the needs of alcohol abusers. Today, over 80 percent of large U.S. firms have EAPs; 31 percent of workers are employed by the nearly 300,000 companies that have EAPs. One reason for this groundswell is our growing acceptance of the Alcoholics Anonymous concept of addiction as a medical illness that requires treatment, not a moral failing. Another reason is that the federal government now requires companies with whom it does business to certify that they are drug-free; the presence of an EAP is one criterion for doing so.

What is an EAP, and what does it do? Basically, EAPs affirm three ideas: Employees are valuable; it's better to assist employees with problems than discipline or fire them; and recovering employees are more productive and effective.

Some companies offer the EAP as an on-site service, as they might provide an employee cafeteria or travel agency. Others —more than half, in fact—contract with EAP providers off the premises.

Wherever it is located, the EAP achieves many goals. It serves as a confidential source of information about treatment for employees and their families. It helps patients make the needed contacts in the company without compromising their position. Importantly, it offers continuing supervision during and after treatment to help the patient remain drug-free. EAPs work for the good of everyone involved. Not only do these programs help those suffering from drug problems, but they lead the fight to increase the use of drug testing, help shape and guide antidrug policy, and contribute to antidrug education in the workplace and in society as a whole. As Barry Feingold predicted in a journal devoted to the EAP movement: "Undoubtedly, the most successful companies in the 1990s and beyond will be those facing the realities of substance abuse by employees and developing policies addressing these concerns."

The people running the EAP are often recovering addicts with formal training in helping others. They need special skills, such as the ability to confront workers with evidence that their work is deteriorating. They must communicate the fact that the employees must be treated before they can return to work. When a company gets this message across loud and clear, employees are more likely to give in and become active participants in the program.

EAPs must have good relationships with hospitals or other facilities and work in harmony with the treatment team of physicians and other health care professionals. The EAP must also support the employee during the course of treatment. This helps workers realize that someone back at the workplace cares enough to take their side and is monitoring their progress.

Knowing they have a job to come back to helps motivate them to participate fully in treatment.

After the employee has been discharged from treatment, the EAP must offer continuing support through individual counseling or group sessions. Many programs require that employees regularly attend Alcoholics Anonymous or Narcotics Anonymous meetings.

A survey of EAPs found that 97 percent of them offer referrals to caregivers or to counselors and that 77 percent offer counseling directly. Over 80 percent make provisions to follow up the patient after treatment. Some EAPs offer telephone hotlines, drug education or awareness programs, and aid for family members. Nine out of ten EAPs are sponsored by company management, and the rest are sponsored by unions or by unions and management in cooperation.

Do EAPs work? Yes. Although statistics can be tricky, some programs can accurately boast a success rate of 75 percent or more. One way that EAPs work is through what we call the "spread of cure." This means that employees return to work after treatment and proselytize about the advantages of the drug-free life.

Don't they cost a lot of money? No, especially when you factor in the savings. For every dollar invested in an EAP, companies save anywhere from $5 to $16 in medical and other costs. For most companies, the average cost of providing such a program works out to about $12 to $20 per employee. Considering the benefits—not the least of which is improved morale—that is money well spent. Another advantage is that they protect companies from legal liability. Less drug use means fewer accidents, disabilities, and deaths.

More good news about EAPs is that as our experience with such programs broadens, so does their effectiveness. Today EAP personnel have their own professional organization that sets standards and accredits programs. Journals devoted to the subject discuss new ways of helping fight drugs in the workplace. The success of the EAP movement means that any company, big or small, can find a program that fits its needs.

Other Solutions Sometimes several companies put their heads together to create an antidrug strategy. For example, thousands of executives have attended conferences organized by the pharmaceutical company Hoffman-LaRoche to discuss the drug problem and share ideas on how to attack it. General Motors and the United Automobile Workers sponsored a 13-week television series broadcast in Detroit that featured recovering substance abusers telling their stories. The Partnership for a Drug-Free America organizes advertising companies and the media to donate their services to create drug "unselling" campaigns.

Recently a number of securities trading firms hammered out a joint pledge to make their industry drug-free. Among the promises made in that pledge were to:

- Implement company drug prevention programs that strive to achieve drug-free workplaces.
- Recognize that drug users may need assistance in overcoming their problems and offer employees with drug problems the opportunity for rehabilitation.
- Distribute written drug policies to all employees, explaining the need to eliminate drug use in the workplace and the individual consequences of such use.
- Require all new hires to sign policy acknowledgments.
- Where permitted by law, test all new hires for illegal drugs.
- Provide Employee Assistance Programs for employees to address drug problems on a confidential basis.
- Train managers to recognize and address drug-related performance problems.
- Communicate with employees about drug policies, EAPs, and program objectives on an ongoing basis.
- Educate our recruiting sources and the community as to the industry position on drug use.

Drug Testing in the Workplace

One of the biggest factors in the rise of drug education and prevention programs is the Drug Free Workplace Act of 1988. This federal legislation requires all companies to certify themselves as providing a drug-free workplace if they receive government grants or if they buy property or services worth more than $25,000 from any federal agency. Other federal guidelines address the controversial issue of drug testing, and I want to end this chapter with a discussion of that vital topic.

The world was stunned when Olympic runner Ben Johnson was stripped of his gold medal after he tested positive for steroids. Some people see such tests as necessary to assure compliance with antidrug policies, whether in sports, business, or any other activity. Others see them as invasions of privacy of the most intimate sort.

What is the truth about drug testing?

First, a little history. Since the 1960s, emergency room physicians have used drug tests to assist in diagnosis and treatment of patients who were comatose, overdosed, or intoxicated. And in the late 1970s, we began using drug tests to help in the psychiatric evaluation of prospective patients. Drug tests could indicate to the physician whether a "manic" patient was really manic or using speed. However, in industry, the idea of screening urine or blood samples for evidence of drug use is relatively new. In fact, a booklet on drug abuse in the workplace published in 1982 by the National Institute of Drug Abuse didn't even mention the term. Drug testing emerged as a strategy in the drug war when the technology became sophisticated enough to assure that results were rapid and accurate, and simple enough for medical technicians to perform without years of training. These developments have occurred only within the last few years. The Greyhound Corporation is generally credited with pioneering the drug-testing movement in the early 1980s. After they launched their program, other companies, including American Airlines, IBM, Burlington Northern

Railroad, Georgia Power Company, Southern Pacific, General Motors, and Exxon did the same.

Though still controversial, drug testing is gaining widespread favor in both the public and the private sectors. In just three years the number of Fortune 500 companies that screened employees for drug use rose from 3 percent to nearly 30 percent. A 1987 survey of a thousand companies by the American Management Association found that 34 percent had a drug-testing policy, up from 21 percent just the year before. In 1988, over 17 million people worked for employers in the private sector that tested for drugs. Nor is support for the battle against drugs limited to executives with their eyes on the bottom line. In a survey of adult workers across the country, over 97 percent said that some form of drug testing at work is appropriate under certain circumstances. More than nine out of ten thought it was a good idea to test pilots and truck drivers.

Why test? A recent study of 2,500 postal employees, published in the *Journal of the American Medical Association,* dramatically illustrates the potential benefits of drug testing. In this study, employees were hired regardless of whether or not they tested positive for drugs. Of the 2,500 new employees, 12 percent tested positive, with marijuana (8 percent of the new hires) and cocaine (2 percent) the most common substances. Those workers who tested positive were at least 50 percent more likely to be fired, injured, disciplined, or absent than those who tested negative. The reasons for drug testing in the workplace vary. As we've seen, some companies implement testing in order to qualify for lucrative government contracts (mercenary, perhaps, but if it cuts down on drug use it's okay by me). Others want to reduce their liability. They don't want their employees involved in accidents for any reason, but especially because they were high on drugs. People who hold jobs that affect public safety, such as airline pilots, surgeons, nurses, bus drivers, police officers, energy workers, and members of the military, need to be especially alert and psychologically stable; use of drugs is a threat to themselves and to others. Still other companies realize the quality of their products is suffering, and so is their business, because of employee drug use.

Whatever the financial and legal reasons behind it, and despite the controversy it engenders, drug testing—used properly and fairly and with all due regard for the individual's civil rights —can identify people in trouble and trigger the process that helps them put their lives back together again. That's perhaps the best feature of drug tests. The sooner we detect substance abuse, the sooner we can begin treatment, and the better the chance that treatment will be successful.

Another benefit of testing is that it acts as a deterrent. Need proof? Before the Coast Guard began testing personnel for drugs, as many as one out of ten members used drugs. Now that testing is part of the routine, only one or two out of a hundred use drugs. The Federal Aviation Administration found even lower rates; only about one half of 1 percent of employees in random tests were found to be drug abusers.

Who tests? Businesses most likely to have testing programs are the mining industry, including oil and gas facilities; communications and public utilities; and transportation industry. As I've noted, some of these companies test in order to comply with regulatory requirements. The least likely to test are retailers, construction companies, and the service industries. One reason is that such companies are more likely to have fewer than ten employees and they usually have a high turnover rate. Widespread testing by the military produced an 82 percent drop in drug use since 1981.

Of those businesses with testing programs, 85 percent test new job applicants (pre-employment testing) and 64 percent focus on current employees (random or annual testing). Most of them test all applicants as one of the final steps before being offered a position. Only 16 percent limited testing to people applying for specific jobs within a company. In those companies that test their employees, two out of three only do so when they suspect a problem with drugs, but one in four tests everybody. In one year, roughly nine workers out of a hundred who work for companies with drug-testing programs—a total of nearly a million people—were actually asked to submit to tests. That's about 1 percent of all workers in the country. Of these, about 9 percent tested positive. Of the 3.9 million job applicants who submitted to tests, 12 percent tested positive—an astonishingly high number considering these applicants knew they were going to be tested. Pre-employment testing identifies users who are in denial or who simply cannot stop taking drugs.

Johnson & Johnson is an example of a large company that tests all applicants for positions. Employees may also be tested if they are involved in accidents or demonstrate unusual behavior. Those in high-risk jobs are tested without advance notice several times a year.

The federal Transportation Department began testing all of its employees in 1988, a move that affected 32,000 workers, mostly air traffic controllers. Starting in late 1989 and continuing through 1990, the department also implemented testing policies that covered nearly four million workers, including aviation personnel, interstate truck drivers, maritime shippers and seamen, railroad workers, employees of companies operating gas pipelines, and urban mass transit workers. The program also calls for random testing of employees in safety-related jobs, as well as testing before employment, after accidents, when drug use is suspected, and at fixed times such as during routine medical exams.

Other government agencies are following suit. The Nuclear Regulatory Commission implemented testing rules in 1989, and recently the Department of Defense demanded that all of its contractors with access to classified information must set up and maintain drug-free workplaces.

Model Programs IBM's approach is often cited as a model for others to follow. "Big Blue" tests all job applicants; if results are positive, they must wait six months before they can reapply. If someone already on the payroll shows a decline in performance, is absent for prolonged periods for unexplained reasons, or shows other erratic behavior, the supervisor reports the problem to the medical department. The employee meets with the company physician and submits to an evaluation including, perhaps, a drug test. Some IBM jobs are considered "safety sensitive"; people in these positions must agree to undergo a test or they will be fired. If test results are positive, the employee enters the assistance program. Before returning to work the employee must be drug-free, take part in a rehabilitation or treatment program, and agree to be monitored by the physician, including periodic, unscheduled urine testing.

What Types of Drug Tests Are Used? *Thin-layer chromatography (TLC)* is a method of separating the molecules of different compounds present in a mixture. The molecules travel to certain points along a plate and stay there. Using special lights, analysts can read the plate and determine the compounds contained in the sample. TLC works best for spotting recent use of drugs in high doses. Because results are notoriously unreliable, positive TLC results need to be confirmed by a more sensitive test.

Immunoassays involve the use of antibodies, which are molecules that attach themselves to an invading substance, such as a drug. In this test, antibodies known to react to illicit drugs are mixed with the urine sample. If a certain antibody—say, the antibody for cocaine—links up with a molecule, the analysts know that the molecule has to be cocaine. Immunoassays are perhaps 100 times more sensitive than TLC. These tests should also be confirmed by a second method.

Gas chromatography, like TLC, separates molecules, but does so using a gas-filled tube rather than a plate. Using an even more refined technique called *mass spectrometry,* labs can break down molecules and determine their exact shape and mass. This test is so accurate—it's a thousand times more sensitive than TLC—that it is considered the equivalent of fingerprinting. It's also expensive, although technological advances are bringing down the costs.

Controversies Concerning Drug Testing

Sometimes labs get wrong results—drugs are present but are not detected (false negative), or they are "detected" but are not present (false positive). For that reason, a positive test must always be confirmed by another and more accurate one. Gas chromatography is far too expensive to be performed routinely as a first screening, but is a virtually foolproof way to confirm the initial results.

Recently, there have been reports of laboratories raising the cutoff level for a positive drug test. A high cutoff level means that employees who are using drugs are not detected (a false negative). Some companies may be going along with this for financial reasons (to avoid using more exact and more expensive tests to confirm or deny the original result) or to avoid legal challenges and controversy. Other companies may be doing this strictly to appear as if they are complying with federal testing requirements. Whatever the reason, if these reports are true, these companies are playing with fire. Ultimately any short-term financial rewards will be dwarfed by increased accidents, employee sick time, theft, and lost productivity.

There are other problems with testing. Marijuana may not show up in a pot smoker's urine for up to four hours. A person may be high as a kite, but if the urine sample is taken within, say, a half hour after toking up, the most accurate test in the world will come up blank. Also, THC can be detected for weeks after the person last smoked. Thus positive results on a lab test may only mean that the person smoked pot sometime within the past month. Cocaine is detectable soon after use, but is usually flushed out of the system within a few days. Thus lab tests for cocaine must be conducted relatively recently after use if they are to be of any help.

Obviously, accuracy is an extremely serious issue. Clerical and other human errors can occur. Employees who have never seen marijuana or who have never been within a hundred miles of cocaine but whose tests produce false positive results will suffer enormously. Not only are their jobs threatened, but they may be stigmatized, wrongly, as drug users. Their careers may be ruined, their lives shattered, all because some bored lab technician mislabeled samples or made an error in calculating the results. This is a very serious and important concern worthy of extra safeguards.

To counteract this problem, the National Institute on Drug Abuse has developed a set of rigid standards a laboratory must meet before it will be allowed to conduct drug tests on government employees. These guidelines cover every possible aspect of the test, from acquisition to storage to analysis to the final report. A chain of custody must be established to assure that the sample never falls into unauthorized hands. Mistakes can still occur, but here is an example of how picky these standards are: In order to qualify for NIDA accreditation, a laboratory has to have a solid ceiling—not a "drop" ceiling that uses foam acoustical tiles. This eliminates the possibility that someone might hide there with the intention of tampering with the samples! The NIDA also conducts "sneak attacks" on labs by sending in samples that are known to be drug-free or that are virtual chemical cocktails. Labs have to score 100 percent on these pop quizzes or they'll lose their contracts. So demanding are these standards that only 33 out of more than 200 laboratories earned the NIDA seal of approval.

Companies have the responsibility to make sure their drug-testing program respects worker's rights, including the right to privacy. Tests must not be conducted arbitrarily or capriciously. Policy has to be communicated clearly to everyone, and the rules have to apply across the board.

I urge that no one should be fired for failing to pass a urine screening. Better to issue a warning for the first offense with an offer for education and rehabilitation. Putting workers on probation gives them the chance to stop using drugs and to enter outpatient or self-help treatment programs. Drug testing should not be considered a weapon, but a means of early detection and a way to prevent the worker from coming to harm.

Many people hear about drug tests and immediately assume that these tests are an invasion of privacy. Lawsuits claim that testing violates the Fourth Amendment, which guarantees freedom from unreasonable search and seizure by the government. Government agencies must weigh these rights against the possible harm to the public that may arise from employee drug abuse. However, private companies are not covered by this amendment, and their decision to test employees does not violate its principle. Indeed, in 1989 the Supreme Court heard two cases, one involving customs employees and the other involving railroad workers. The court ruled that public safety outweighs the right of individuals to privacy, thus upholding the practice of drug tests in these cases.

Often, legal challenges to drug testing focus on the use of random tests. Opponents feel random tests violate individual rights. However, in 1989 lower courts ruled in favor of random testing in five cases involving police officers, prison guards, Justice Department employees with top secret security clearances, and nuclear plant workers. If these cases are argued all the way to the Supreme Court, the rulings are likely to be upheld.

Leadership

A company's role in the war against drugs involves more than drug-testing programs, EAPs, and drug education programs. A company that actively confronts the drug abuse problem in its workforce sends an invaluable message to its workers, their families, their communities, and their schools: *Drug abuse will not and cannot be tolerated.* In short, a company's role involves leadership.

I can think of no finer example of corporate leadership than the Partnership for a Drug-Free America. As I explained earlier, the Partnership is an alliance of media and advertising executives dedicated to using the latest advertising and marketing skills in the war against drugs. These individuals, with the support of their companies, have taken a stand against drugs, and our country has benefited enormously from their efforts.

Many of the Partnership initial ads have been targeted at the occasional drug user, i.e., the drug user most likely to be employed and the one most likely to benefit from early intervention. As I have stated on numerous occasions, the single greatest form of treatment is prevention. Employees who know that their company is concerned about drug use are less likely to experiment with drugs. Drug abuse is a disease that depends upon its victim to take the first step. Without that first step, there is no disease. As more and more companies take an open stand against drugs, American attitudes against drugs become stronger and the tolerant atmosphere that allows drug use to foster disappears.

CHAPTER TWELVE

In Our Society

Washington D.C.: As part of his Drug Control Strategy, President Bush announces he will make available over a billion dollars a year for drug prevention and education, an increase of 25 percent over the previous year. He also increases funds for treatment by 53 percent, to a record level of nearly a billion dollars.

Seattle: Cops attack drug dealers using the latest weapon in the drug war: mountain bicycles. Drug-pushing gang members who once laughed at the sight of their opponents on bicycles aren't laughing anymore; after some impressive arrests, open drug dealing has fallen off. The "bike guys" are now perceived as the toughest cops on the beat.

San Francisco: Alarmed at the presence of a crack house in their neighborhood, and frustrated at the city's bureaucratic inertia, residents lay siege to the house's owners. Their tactic: a barrage of lawsuits filed in small claims court. Though the amount of each claim is small, the total impact is tremendous: The drug dealers are routed, and the residents reclaim their neighborhood as their own.

At every level of our society, from the federal down to the

grass-roots, people are mobilizing to tackle the drug problem. As the examples above show, the solutions they devise are ingenious and resourceful. And these solutions work.

Strategy at the National Level

In September of 1989 President Bush announced his plan for controlling drugs. His strategy expanded on steps taken by Ronald Reagan, who a few years earlier convened the White House Conference for a Drug-Free America. I had the privilege of serving as an adviser on both of these projects.

I wasn't alone—our national leaders assembled an extraordinary team, made up not just of high-level experts but ordinary concerned citizens as well. This team took a hard look at drug use in this country, recognized its gravity, and created a blueprint to bring the problem under control. These leaders have taken their cue from American citizens who have risen up in opposition to the drugs in their own streets and neighborhoods. Their success stories, some of which I'll report in this chapter, clearly indicate that the war against drugs is a guerrilla war to be fought and won on the doorsteps and in the alleyways of our country.

Bush titled his plan the *National Drug Control Strategy.* Critics claimed that by emphasizing control over drugs and not their elimination, the administration had admitted defeat before the war had begun. This criticism, while somewhat understandable, fails to address the real source of America's drug problem.

A policy that focuses on control attacks the problem while honoring the American concept of civil rights. (Even notorious drug lord Manuel Noriega was promised a fair trial.) It also recognizes that while we may commit vast resources to the fight, there will always be limits to those resources. The strategy of control is realistic; being realistic, it has a much greater chance of success. As Yale professor David F. Musto observes, stressing total elimination at this stage of the game would blind us to intermediate measures that will do a better job of helping people kick the habit—or, better yet, keeping them from developing a habit in the first place.

The Bush plan stresses the need to reduce the level of drug use along its entire spectrum: experimental first use, casual use, and addiction. With this as its highest priority, the plan recognizes that reducing the demand for drugs is a more effective approach than reducing supply. The strategy for the first two years is to cut in half the rate of increase in the number of people who use cocaine once a week or more. A modest goal—perhaps too modest, given the already stunning decline in cocaine use we saw beginning in the late 1980s. Over ten years, however, the goal is to reduce the actual number of weekly coke users by 50 percent. A tougher challenge, but one I know we can meet.

Bennett named Dr. Herbert D. Kleber as his deputy for demand reduction. Dr. Kleber and I have known each other for many years—the government's strategy couldn't be in more capable hands. When a reporter asked Dr. Kleber how the goal will be achieved, he replied, "We will not only work harder but work smarter."

Reducing demand means educating people about drugs. Thirty percent of the entire drug-control budget, representing a 36 percent increase over previous antidrug plans, is earmarked for education, prevention, and treatment. In addition, the Secretary of Education has pledged funds to create antidrug videotapes, parents' handbooks, and other educational programs.

The Bush plan also provides federal support for local drug prevention efforts, antidrug media events, and efforts to guarantee drug-free workplaces. One strategy requires that schools, including universities, set up prevention programs before they are eligible to receive federal funds. The underlying goal is to create within our society the attitude that drug use is unacceptable.

Importantly, the plan identifies ways to better treat people with drug problems. In its call for a responsible and compassionate policy, the plan targets certain groups who most need help, such as expectant mothers. There is more money available to create not just new openings in treatment facilities, but new methods of treatment as well, a subject dear to my own heart. To reach that goal, the plan calls for improvements in research, both in the lab and in the clinic. Steps toward that goal include creating a national drug database, studying the nature of addiction, examining treatment success rates, and developing new technologies for use against illegal drugs.

The rest of the money will go for law enforcement, including interdiction and corrections, for example. Of course, we need these other elements. Too often drug dealers think they can, literally, get away with murder and still incur no punishment. The Bush plan calls for stiffer penalties and shores up the criminal justice system at every point, from arrest through prosecution to rehabilitation after release from jail. Another approach that will help is tightening up the restrictions on the sale of the chemicals that are used to make illegal drugs. Thus a drug dealer who has to buy the ether needed to produce cocaine, for example, would leave a paper trail, making it much easier for drug agency officers to track him down.

The National Strategy also supports the notion of drug testing when appropriate. I discussed the value of drug tests in the previous chapter and won't dwell on the subject here. Briefly, though, drug testing is a powerful deterrent, an excellent way of identifying people who need treatment, and essential for monitoring the success of treatment.

Although the Strategy places emphasis on the home front, it also provides nearly half a billion dollars to wage war at the international level. The weapons in our international arsenal include eradication, interdiction, and extradition. Recently there's been a big change in other countries' attitudes. Before, they felt that drug use was an American problem; as long as there were rich gringos willing to blow their life savings, not to mention their minds, on drugs, well, they were there to supply them. But now these countries admit that the problem exists in their own backyards. Colombia has about 500,000 regular cocaine smokers—more addicts per capita than the United States.

Burma has 300,000 heroin and opium addicts. Other Asian countries must deal with thousands of citizens who use ice and other drugs.

Some progress has been made due to our efforts to eradicate drug crops with the cooperation of foreign nations. As recent headlines show, eradication reduces the supply of drugs and makes it harder for drug thugs to stay in business. A few years ago, for example, we put a significant kink in the drug pipeline when we wiped out nearly 5 percent of Bolivia's coca fields.

Interdiction means seizing drugs before they reach the market. Stopping ships loaded with cocaine or airplanes crammed with bales of marijuana interrupts supply, raising the street price of drugs and thus curtailing purchases. Also, when drug dealers feel the heat, and when their regular supply routes and contacts are cut off, they have to create new ones and risk exposing themselves and their operations.

Another powerful weapon is extradition—the legal right to bring foreign criminals to trial in our country. Drug lords—*narcotraficantes,* as they are known in Latin America—truly fear extradition. As one said, "We prefer a Colombian grave to an American jail." Greater international cooperation has made extradition an even bigger threat.

Of course, no plan is perfect. Although the National Drug Control Strategy is the most comprehensive and well-supported antidrug effort in the nation's history, there will always be those who claim that this plan doesn't go far enough. Often, their criticisms are valid.

I, too, would like to see more money spent on treatment, drug education, and research. I would also like to see specific plans targeted at the few remaining areas where drugs continue to be a problem—our cities. In Chapter One, I presented my plan for confronting these troublesome areas.

State and Local Strategies

National policy sets the pace for action at the state and local level. New Jersey is often cited as a model of a tough antidrug stance. Let me describe how it earned its reputation.

Tough Laws The state's Comprehensive Drug Reform Act, which took effect in July 1987, is based, like the Bush plan, on the idea that cutting off supply isn't enough; we must also reduce demand. One way is through deterrence. To deter drug use, the state sends out the message that all drug offenders, including users, are accountable for their actions. Offenders realize that not only are they likely to get caught, they also will suffer meaningful punishment when they are. Punishment, however, is structured such that offenders are guided toward rehabilitation and treatment programs. Much of the focus in New Jersey is on the need to make the schools drug-free centers for learning, rather than handy outlets for dealers and users.

The state penalties for drug offenses are clearly spelled out. For example, all drug offenders encounter mandatory cash fines; wisely, the money collected is channeled into community programs designed to further reduce demand. So far millions of dollars taken from drug offenders' pockets have gone to support prevention, education, and public awareness programs. I love imagining that one day all such programs will begin with the announcement: "Brought to you by a grant from your local pushers and addicts."

All people convicted of drug offenses in the state automatically lose their driver's licenses for at least six months to two years. In 1988 alone nearly 10,000 licenses were suspended. And get this—the suspension doesn't *begin* until the offender turns 17. For a 14-year-old kid to realize that he won't be able to drive for five more years if he is caught with drugs can have real impact on his choice to use drugs. At that age, five years seems like an eternity.

Schools The marrow of the New Jersey antidrug policy, and one of its most visible and successful elements, is its drug-free school zone strategy. Community leaders literally sit down with a map and draw a circle around each school—public, private, parochial. The circle (usually with a thousand-foot radius, but in Alabama, with a radius of three miles) indicates a zone of protection. Distinctive blue-and-white signs indicate the boundaries of those zones to all who enter them. Any person committing a drug offense within this radius is subject to even harsher penalties than elsewhere in the community. For starters, offenders are given an automatic three-year trip to jail—no questions asked, no possibility of parole. The drug-free zone policy also sets up clear guidelines for police officers, guidelines that govern arrests, searches, seizures, undercover operations, and patrols of school grounds and activities. The policy also spells out the teachers' role in confiscating drugs and turning students suspected of drug crimes over to police.

After just a few years, it has become clear that the drug-free school-zone strategy promotes a healthier environment in which kids can learn and teachers can teach. At the same time it helps the students understand the pressure they are under to use drugs, and gives them the support they need to resist.

A year after New Jersey's drug-free school zone program was launched, Congress passed a similar law at the federal level. To be effective, however, each state must follow New Jersey's lead in enacting tough legislation that empowers its police to enforce the antidrug policy within those zones.

The impact of the policy has had a carryover effect. For example, laws that prohibit liquor stores within half a mile of schools have resulted in fewer serious problems with alcohol. Similarly, tougher laws against selling tobacco to minors have reduced the rate of cigarette smoking and, indirectly, the dency for kids using this gateway drug to go on and develop other drug habits, such as smoking marijuana or crack.

Police Strong law enforcement is crucial if drug laws are to have any teeth. In New Jersey, police departments are instructed that enforcing the drug laws and the policy of Zero Tolerance is their number one priority. Officers arrest *all* drug offenders, regardless of the quantity of drugs involved.

Earlier I mentioned Seattle's innovative approach to law enforcement: an antidrug patrol mounted on bicycles. Phoenix, Arizona, has also had great success with a new drug policy that focuses on the casual user and is thought by some to be the toughest big-city drug crackdown in America. Police patrol nightspots and parks and arrest anyone they catch using drugs; sometimes the arrests are made under the glare of TV lights and cameras—the kind of publicity that no one wants. The policy is marketed to citizens through its copyrighted slogan, "Do drugs—do time." Other posters show hands shackled with handcuffs and bear the headline, "What the casual drug user will be wearing this season." One significant part of the crackdown's success has been its innovative penalty system. After their first night in jail, offenders are given a choice: face felony charges or enter a drug-treatment program. Most choose treatment, and must pay for each urine test until they prove clean. They also have to pay for a six-hour antimarijuana lecture, and chip in $500 to reimburse the town for police and court costs. Cocaine users have it rougher; their program lasts up to two years and costs them nearly $3,000. So effective is Phoenix's strategy of "user accountability" that its police chief, Ruben B. Ortega, was named to William Bennett's advisory panel, and continues to serve under Bob Martinez.

Recently the National Association of Chiefs of Police kicked off a campaign called Going Straight: Toward a Drug-free America. The program, aimed at reducing demand for drugs, brings together law enforcement, parents, educators, and community and private sector leaders to promote education, prevention, and enforcement.

Having a police force active in enforcement sends a very visible signal about society's attitude toward drugs. What's more, police patrols make it harder for drug users to gain access to their suppliers, raising both the cost and the time involved in making the buy. As Mark Kleiman, a lecturer on criminal justice at Harvard, notes, "If you are a heavy user and the probability of not connecting is great, that becomes a strong argument for getting into a treatment program."

Other Solutions Some states and communities have come up with some highly creative ways of solving the drug problem in their areas. Since 1986, Minnesota, Illinois, Nevada, Texas, and Kansas have imposed drug stamp taxes. Dealers in those states must buy tax stamps according to the drug and its weight. Pot dealers, for example, have to buy (anonymously and confidentially) a $5 stamp for every gram of marijuana they intend to sell. If they are caught selling the drug without that stamp, they can be prosecuted for tax violations as well as drug violations. (In this country, it is possible to tax an activity even though it is illegal.) Within three years, dealers had already been assessed fines for "back taxes" totalling more than $50 million! Dealers are motivated to buy the stamps because doing so is better than risking the penalties for failure to comply. The vast amounts of money collected can be used to pay for more treatment centers and police.

As we saw with the Phoenix approach, users are charged for the costs of their prosecution and treatment. Recently a University of Iowa student was convicted of distributing LSD. The judge in that case ordered him to pay "rent" of $1,210 per month for his stay in prison. After his release he must also pay $91 a month for four years of supervision. Programs that hit drug users where they live—in their wallets—take some of the heat off our overburdened courts, prisons, and treatment facilities and place the responsibility where it belongs: on the offender.

California has implemented the "Civil Addict Program," in which those convicted of drug offenses are sent to treatment facilities instead of, or in addition to, incarceration. Those in the program are closely monitored, which means, among other things, frequent urine tests and the threat of going back to jail after a positive test. Studies show that involuntary treatment works just as well as the voluntary kind, and in the future we may see more states requiring users to enter a therapy program rather than making it an option.

Another strategy that works: Confiscate from drug dealers their drug profits and property—cars, houses, boats—that was bought with proceeds from their illegal trafficking. There is already a law permitting such seizures in federal cases; 17 states have similar laws. The policy works partly because it requires the dealer to prove that the possessions *weren't* bought with drug money. In all, 39 states allow authorities to seize the cash resulting from drug sales, and more state legislatures are considering passing or broadening such laws.

Social Strategies

Many of the tactics I've described so far in this chapter rely on legal action by our national, state, and local governments. But there's a lot that we as individual citizens can do. We've already talked about steps parents can take in their own homes, even before their children are born, to create a loving atmosphere that helps inoculate against drug use. And of course, any effort we as a society can make to reduce poverty, joblessness, and illiteracy will help keep our kids away from drugs.

Those of you who are old enough to remember the Surgeon General's anticigarette proclamations of the early 1960s have seen how government leadership can influence social actions. It didn't happen overnight; several years passed before the effects of the antismoking campaign could be assessed. In 1960, there were over 50 million smokers, 25 years later that number had been reduced to 38 million (although our overall population increased significantly during that time). Not only did the antismoking campaign greatly reduce the number of smokers, it has had a surprising effect upon our social behavior. The knowledge that smoking, even passive inhalation of another person's smoke, could harm people led to health-conscious citizens demanding changes. Thirty years ago very few people would have ever predicted smoke-free offices, airplane flights, and hotel rooms. Today, smoking has such a negative image that smokers have complained of being treated as second-class citizens.

Like the antismoking campaign, the war against drugs is a

battle of inches. Our greatest hope comes from the actions of individual people. As Jacob V. Lamar commented in *Time* magazine, any glimmer of hope we have "comes from the social workers, the community activists and Samaritans who are reaching out to children, one by one, trying to give them the affection and guidance that may keep them from surrendering their lives" to drugs. My files are full of examples of these grassroots successes.

New Jersey: Inspired by the success of the drug-free school zones, the state assembly passed a bill authorizing neighborhoods to declare themselves "drug-free block zones." Yellow signs announcing the fact would indicate areas where stiffer-than-usual drug penalties would be enforced. Said Robert C. Shinn, the assemblyman who sponsored the measure, "The war on drugs must be won, even if we have to fight it a block at a time."

Pennsylvania: Nearly 600 utility workers in 41 counties in the state have been trained to spot signs of illegal drug activities in rural areas and to notify police when they suspect something is amiss. Rural electric workers who travel the back roads are in a position to recognize the signs that a clandestine drug lab, such as one that makes methamphetamines, is operating in the area. Clues include chemical odors, discarded chemical containers, fans whirring through the night, high consumption of water or electricity, and extreme fluctuations in power use. Drug makers like to choose out-of-the-way spots for their operations so that they won't have neighbors breathing down their necks or complaining about noise or fumes. Inspired by the Pennsylvania program, and believing that utility companies have a role in solving the growing drug problem in rural America, the National Rural Electric Cooperative Association is developing a national program along similar lines.

Providence, R.I.: The Elmwood Neighbors for Action operate car patrols to intimidate potential drug buyers. When they spot a sale in progress, members use their car phones—supplied by the state—to report details to police.

Los Angeles: A group calling itself the Beat Keepers has

Fighting Back: Profiles from the War on Drug's Hall of Fame

Robert Armstrong

Position: Director of the Omaha, Nebraska, Housing Authority.

Achievements: Evicted known drug pushers from public housing. Worked with schools to allow dropouts to return more quickly; launched academic incentive awards and scholarship programs for high school students in public housing; organized a cleanup campaign. Fostered cooperation between residents and police.

Quote: "This is no time for despair. We can't give up. Each of us needs to accept our responsibility to get totally involved."

Erma Scales

Position: Volunteer chair of the Acres Homes War on Drugs Committee, Houston, Texas.

Achievements: Formed a neighborhood watch program, writing down license plates and turning in dealers to police. Tore down abandoned buildings used as crack houses and cleared vacant lots of high brush that concealed drug deals. Organized a group to march on a local park and wrested it away from dealers. Created a comprehensive antidrug program—education, treatment, neighborhood patrols, drug-free activity for young people—using business donations.

Quote: "We need to teach our system of values. Parents need to spend more time with their kids and go back to being parents."

Alvin Brooks

Position: Founder of the Ad Hoc Group Against Crime, Kansas City, Missouri.

Achievements: Set up 24-hour Youth Information and Drug Abuse Hotline. Pressured stores to stop selling drug paraphernalia. Founded Black Men Together to offer role models to young people; members take youngsters to sports events and on tours of courts and prisons, hold

Continued

antidrug seminars in schools, help young people find jobs. They patrol streets with bullhorns, warning them, "Hey you, dope dealer, black men out here are watching you."

Quote: "Just our presence causes drug pushers to leave the area. We stand like men, act like men, and we're respected like men."

Margaret Toomey

Position: Founder of project HOPE (Homes of Oakridge Prevention Effort), Des Moines, Iowa.

Achievements: Organized tenants to work against drugs, evicting 60 families involved in dealing. Sponsored programs to alert youth to dangers of drugs. Created the Inner City Single Parent Vocational Program to help people become self-sufficient.

Quote: "Stand up and be counted. Do it cautiously, do it carefully—but do it."

adopted a battlecry: "Beat the crack and take the neighborhood back!" The group's tactic—not one I recommend to everyone—is to confront the dealers that had taken over the corner of Hollywood and Vine and harass them into leaving the area.

Detroit: A mother of two, horrified as warring drug dealers shot up a house a block away, organized a march in protest. During the march the troupe, carrying signs made from materials donated by local merchants, came upon a dealer about to make a sale. They did nothing more than stare at the dealer, who, seeing he was surrounded, disappeared.

To acknowledge such grass-roots efforts, and to encourage others to follow their example, William Bennett recognized individuals and groups in a program he called "Fighting Back." For a summary of some of these success stories, see the Box on pages 240–41.

As you see, there is virtually no end to the power one person has, or to the ways that power can be used. The secret—no secret at all, really—is to establish the goal, communicate that goal one person at a time, and organize the resources needed to meet that goal.

Another key strategy is to realize that those who most need to hear the message may be those who are hardest to reach. Dropouts, for example, are in no position to benefit from a school program. To reach them you have to find them. That takes a blend of skill, stamina, and a healthy helping of street savvy. Many grass-roots strategists know that peers have an enormous amount of influence. Recruiting teenagers to talk to teenagers can make all the difference.

Don't overlook other sources of help. As we saw, the Detroit marchers got local merchants to donate poster board and wood to make signs for their march. Churches can become involved, not just through the counseling services of the clergy but by donating use of their facilities for community rallies or Narcotics Anonymous meetings. Librarians can supply lists of materials—books, videotapes, recordings—to create a community database for use against drugs. Local residents with special expertise—nurses, fundraisers, writers, and so on—are usually willing and proud to offer their skills. I do what I can to encourage my fellow physicians to become involved, and to share their antidrug expertise with parents and community groups.

Often kids who have tuned out the antidrug messages from their parents or teachers will pay attention when someone special speaks to them. Drew Brown, the first black man to pilot a Navy attack jet, reaches students by showing up in his blue-and-yellow pilot's uniform and speaking in a blunt, no-nonsense way. Sure, he tells his eager listeners, everybody wants to be happy and have fun. But the harder you work, the higher your level of fun. Citing his own success, he says, "Since I went to college my level of fun is high. When I party, I party in Paris. When I jam, I jam in Jamaica." Pulling no punches, he tells kids: "You better wake up. I know some of you don't want to listen. You're too bad to listen to me. But that's okay, because when I pull into the McDonald's drive-through in my black Cadillac, I'm going to need you to hand me my large fries."

Grass-roots efforts work best when they ally with local law enforcement officials who can work with residents to implement their plans. Police officers make a big impression; showing kids that behind the badges and the guns are people who genuinely care about their health and safety can make the difference in their attitudes toward the law.

Kids need role models. Many grass-roots groups make an effort to recognize young people who exemplify the positive aspects of a drug-free life. Doing so reinforces their efforts, and makes them feel part of a larger drug-free community. It also shows the others that it is indeed possible to resist pressure, and that success comes to those who stay clean. As the report announcing Bush's National Drug Control Strategy states, "In the war against illegal drug use, the real heroes are not those who use drugs and quit; they are those who never use them in the first place."

Dramatically, in his school appearances, Drew Brown calls out the names of honor roll students and asks them to stand up. "If you want to see 'bad,' look around you because they are the real role models. I hear some of you laughing, and I know some of you think they are nerds, but in 10, 15 years, they'll have big nerdy houses and big nerdy cars. And all you people who think you're 'bad' will be asking, 'Excuse me, sir? Do I get out of this prison in 10 years, or is it 15?' "

According to a *Wall Street Journal* poll, two out of three voters believe that movies, television, and music stimulate people to try drugs. Recently the media—advertising, television, movies—have taken steps to respond to such criticism by promoting the antidrug message. Earlier I mentioned the Partnership for a Drug-Free America, which creates and distributes antidrug commercials—the largest single advertising effort ever undertaken in the United States, and entirely voluntary. Perhaps their most effective ad so far shows an egg as a voice intones, "This is your brain." The egg is cracked into a sizzling frying pan; the voice says, "This is your brain on drugs." Marketing researchers have proved that people who see these ads change their attitudes about drugs. I think this approach is terrific. For the first time, we are seeing advertising used as a form of medical intervention—a form of preventive health care distributed over the airwaves.

The Partnership spots don't use celebrities to get their message across. Another group, the Entertainment Industries Council, does produce antidrug ads featuring celebrities. If these messages reach kids and make a difference in their lives, then fine. But I suspect that antidrug commercials with sports figures and rock stars who are reformed drug users may send the wrong message: "Look at me! I used drugs—not only did I survive, I'm still rich and successful." I prefer hearing from antidrug spokespeople like Drew Brown who stayed clean and still made it to the top.

More good news: All three major networks now have drug censors on staff to make sure the message is clear. Scripts featuring people involved in drugs must show those people coming to bad ends because of their drug use. Shows such as *Saturday Night Live* can't get away with sketches showing drugs as a source of fun and frolic. Similarly, the Caucus for Producers, Writers, and Directors has drafted a position paper that opposes the glamorous portrayal of drugs and alcohol in the media.

We need to make more progress in this area, though. So many sports activities are sponsored by makers of beer and cigarettes that viewers get the confusing message that these products are part and parcel of the healthy, active lifestyle. Recently one distiller sponsored a "frequent drinker" promotion: Airline passengers who sent in labels from the bottles they bought in-flight would receive free upgrades to first-class tickets or discounts on merchandise. Phooey! We don't need to give people incentives to drink! Perhaps the new warning labels on liquor containers will help. I also applaud the liquor industry's sponsorship of messages promoting more responsible drinking. One recent ad for Coors beer, for example, put a nice spin on its slogan, "It's the right beer now"; the ad shows people hunting or about to get into their cars, and the announcer says—forcefully—"But not now." If we can't eliminate liquor or its advertisements completely, this is at least a trend in the right direction.

Legalization

Before I close this chapter, I want to comment on a recurring social movement that could undo all the progress we have made against drugs over the last two decades: the legalization of drugs.

By now, you can probably guess my position on the issue. I'm against it. But, with the violence and frustration drugs cause in our cities, legalization will continue to be an issue for the 1990s. Let me explain why. To do so I have to state the other side's point of view. Having admitted my prejudice, then, I'll do my best to frame the issues in the debate.

Basically, proponents of legalization argue that by removing criminal penalties for drug sale and use we will unclog our courts, stop the black market for drugs, empty our jails, free our police officers to focus on other crimes, and use the money we save to promote treatment. As the government steps in to regulate the industry the way it now does alcohol, we can tax drugs, raise oodles of revenue, control quality, lower the prices, and drive the illegal dealers out of business. With the profit motive gone, dealers will have to find something else to do with their marketing skills. And given enough time, users will learn moderation.

Bull.

Legalization advocates often point to the example of Prohibition, which, they claim, failed to eliminate the human tendency to chemically alter our state of consciousness. So strong was our desire to intoxicate ourselves, they point out, that Prohibition was repealed a few years after its passage.

Failed? Look again: During the Prohibition era, alcohol use dropped by 30 to 50 percent. Deaths from cirrhosis of the liver fell from 29.5 per 100,000 in 1911 to 10.7 in 1929. Admissions to state mental hospitals for alcohol psychosis fell from 10.1 per 100,000 in 1919 to 4.7 in 1928. According to Mark Moore, Harvard professor of criminal justice, Prohibition *succeeded:* It reduced by one third the consumption of a drug that had been widely used for thousands of years. In his editorial in *The New York Times,* Moore wrote: "The real lesson of Prohibition is that the society can, indeed, make a dent in the consumption of drugs through laws." He concludes, "The common claim that laws backed by morally motivated political movements cannot reduce drug use is wrong. . . . If the line is held now, we can prevent new [drug] users and increasing casualties. So this is exactly *not* the time to be considering a liberalization of our laws [on drugs]. . . ." To that I say, Amen.

How did this subject even come up? Why, after years of fighting the drug wars, are some people considering throwing in the towel?

One spark that reignited the issue came in 1988 when the eloquent Baltimore mayor Kurt Schmoke grabbed headlines by urging a national debate on legalization. His charismatic argument focused on his career as a prosecutor and on his frustration with current antidrug efforts. He pointed out just how profitable drugs are; remove the profit motive, and you put the dealers out of business. In Schmoke's view, we might be able to walk into government stores, much like liquor stores, and buy packages of marijuana cigarettes—all nicely wrapped, purity and potency guaranteed, complete with cellophane wrap and a cute little tax stamp signifying government approval. But could we advertise these officially approved products on TV? Could we buy drug products like PCP? Could addicts register with the public health system to qualify for clean needles? Would crack be available daily, or would we give a weekly supply?

After Schmoke's initial speech, several national figures jumped on the legalization bandwagon, including the conservative columnist William F. Buckley; George Shultz, Reagan's secretary of state; Milton Friedman, Nobel Prize–winning economist; and Ira Glasser, head of the American Civil Liberties Union. Many of these high-ranking individuals credit (I would prefer the word "blame") Ethan A. Nadelmann, a teacher at the Woodrow Wilson School of Public and International Affairs at Princeton University, for convincing them to at least consider legalization. Some advocates want to legalize all drugs; others limit the debate to the legalization of marijuana only.

In late 1989, a federal judge, Robert W. Sweet, became the first person in his position to propose legalization. Judge Sweet argued that illicit drugs should be treated like alcohol: taxed, made illegal for minors, banned from the workplace, etc. He proposed nothing that others hadn't suggested, but got the nation's attention because as a judge he was perceived as someone who was supposed to enforce the laws against drugs.

As a drug treatment specialist, I feel like a soldier on the front lines. People who advocate legalization want to take away our guns and our bullets when we are winning the war. They ignore the millions of current users and leave us defenseless against the onslaught of addiction that would overwhelm us without legal sanctions against drugs.

It makes no sense—medically, socially, or ethically—to quit just when we are making tremendous headway against drugs. While legalization might help Judge Sweet clear his docket to deal with what he considers more pressing cases, it would make it possible for even more people to get their hands on drugs, become addicts, and cause the currently half-empty treatment facilities to fill again. Experts predict that with legalization, we could be faced with perhaps 12 million new addicts, in addition to the millions we already have to contend with. In the words of the editorialists for *The New York Times,* legalizing cocaine is a crack-brained idea.

Legalization advocates ignore the fact that drug use is kept to a certain level because it is hard, costly, and illegal to obtain drugs. Does anyone honestly believe that drug use will decline if people can just walk into the local 7-Eleven and pick up a 20-pack of reefers or a bag of cocaine, along with their chips and Pepsi?

"Oh, but legalization would reduce crime," they argue. Okay, some addicts may commit fewer crimes to pay for their habits. But addicts use drugs as often as they can. Less-expensive, easily obtainable drugs means they'll use them more often—and they'll *still* need to cough up the cash to make their buys. And more use of drugs means more side effects like paranoia, irritability, and violence. With legal crack we might have fewer robberies, but more assaults, murders, more addicts, more overdoses, more deaths, more need for treatment, and higher health costs. It's a trade-off, not a solution, and it ain't worth it, folks.

Besides, many addicts are criminals anyway. Even if they didn't rob old ladies to pay for drugs, they'd rob old ladies to pay for food. According to Dr. Mitchell S. Rosenthal, an expert on drugs and adolescents and president of Phoenix House, a resident treatment center in New York: "If you give somebody free drugs you don't turn him into a responsible employee, husband, or father."

"But marijuana addiction is no worse than alcohol addiction." Who needs another social problem on the same scale as alcoholism? Not I, said the doctor.

"Legal drugs would lower prices and eliminate the profits from illegal drug trafficking, and drive drug lords out of business." In order to undercut the drug cartels, the government would have to price its cocaine at about $10 per gram—50 cents a dose, or roughly the price of a Snickers candy bar. That puts it within the budget of every kid in America. Besides, if the government-approved product were of lower quality or potency than the black-market variety, people would *still* buy from illegal sources to reach the high they seek.

"Taxing drugs would raise funds for treatment." But if you didn't make it so easy for people to become addicted, you wouldn't need to treat them in the first place, would you!

There is another point that legalization supporters conveniently ignore: Namely, drugs run in cycles. Historically, a period where stimulants (i.e., cocaine) are popular is usually followed by an era when use of depressants (i.e., heroin) increases, which in turn is followed by another stimulant era. Would the laws governing legalization have to be constantly amended to allow for these changing patterns of use? And consider the ever-enterprising basement chemists: Would any legalization laws have to allow for the advent of new drugs similar to the ice and ecstasy of the 1980s? Legalization isn't the answer, it only raises more difficult questions.

I see good news in the results of surveys showing that as

many as eight out of nine Americans oppose legalization. Perhaps I should place more trust in the power of good ol' common sense to prevail. Meanwhile, I continue to hope that the debate will merely expose the fallacies of the arguments in its favor and will strengthen the merits of continuing our fight against drugs through prevention, education, and treatment.

CHAPTER THIRTEEN

Medical Research Works

Medicine: the only profession that labours
incessantly to destroy the reason
for its existence.
—*James Bryce*
(British diplomat, 1838–1922)

If I could invent a pill that would cure all drug users of their addiction, even if it meant that my work in the substance abuse treatment field would end, I would be ecstatic. Part of the good news is that, over the past two decades, some powerful medications have indeed emerged that enable many addicts to take further steps along on their road to recovery. In this chapter I'll describe those medications and some of the other breakthroughs developed in medical research labs.

Medical Treatment of Cocaine Addiction

"Once, in college, I took part in a hunger strike," a patient named Hilary told me. "I held out for seven days. But the hunger I felt then was *nothing* compared to the hunger I feel if I don't have cocaine."

Hilary was describing the craving that her coke addiction produced. In the battle against the White Devil, the craving is our wiliest enemy. I've mentioned this before, but it bears repeating: So strong is the craving that laboratory animals, allowed free access to cocaine, will continue to self-administer cocaine until it kills them.

The craving can be so strong that it may prevent users from even considering treatment. They can't imagine doing without their precious drug. Often cravings cause patients to drop out of treatment—sometimes escaping from the hospital in the dead of night—because they can't hold out during the detoxification period.

Cravings emerge in different forms during the different stages of cocaine use and withdrawal. Immediately following a cocaine binge, users experience a crash marked by severe depression, agitation, and anxiety. Often users interpret these feelings to mean they must take more of the drug. Oddly, though, during the four-hour period following the binge, the craving for cocaine may actually be overwhelmed by the craving for sleep. Because cocaine is a stimulant, users may not be able to sleep, and so they turn to sedative drugs—anything from alcohol to marijuana to opiates to sleeping pills—to put them under. For one to four days coke bingers suffer a form of hangover marked by periods of extreme sleepiness, ravenous appetite, and lousy moods.

The next type of craving emerges during withdrawal. At Fair Oaks, Don Sweeney, Charles Dackis, and I studied the powerful effects of that craving or even the memory of a high can have during withdrawal. Talcum powder, fake cocaine, or even pictures of cocaine can produce such strong feelings that ex-users have asked to be locked up! The symptoms of withdrawal from cocaine are the mirror image of the drug's effects: decreased energy, lack of interest in anything, and an inability to feel pleasure. These symptoms increase and fluctuate in intensity over the four days following a binge. However, the contrast between the high of cocaine use and the low of withdrawal is so strong that it induces the craving and impels the user to another binge. Thus the cycle begins again; thus spins the Wheel of Misfortune. It can take an individual user as long as four months of total abstinence before they feel the symptoms of withdrawal disappear. Four months is a very long time; most addicts can't hold out that long without some kind of help—or without returning to the drug.

Even if they do manage to quit, there's always the threat that the cravings will recur. I've handled cases where patients felt overwhelming coke cravings up to *seven years* after their last snort. During this stage cravings can be triggered by just about anything—the sight of snow, or sugar, or talcum powder; a song; the recurrence of a certain mood; the voice of a person the user associates with drug use; visiting the site of former coke experiences. One patient told me that on a camping trip he was trying to shave using a small hand-mirror; just handling the mirror caused his craving to erupt after five years of abstinence, and he cut his trip short to go search for the drug. New research on the neuroanatomy and chemistry of craving may help explain this phenomenon and its power over the individual. (See the discussion of kindling in Chapter Seven.) In the meantime, a goal of treatment is to counsel patients to deal with these triggers and remain abstinent. We all have desires or cravings, yet we do not act on them. We know for a fact that in time, and with continued abstinence, the cravings will diminish in intensity until eventually they will be extinguished. You can, of course, have all kinds of cravings and never act on them.

Earlier I described how cocaine depletes the brain of the neurotransmitter dopamine, first by stimulating cells to secrete the chemical and then by blocking its reabsorption so that it eventually is washed away in the bloodstream. Without enough dopamine, the user experiences the symptoms of withdrawal I've just described.

The good news: A medication exists that does a pretty good job of removing the initial cravings associated with stopping cocaine use. That medication is bromocriptine.

Bromocriptine, sold under the brand name Parlodel and used as a treatment for Parkinson's disease, absence of menstruation, and other disorders, works in part by stimulating the dopamine receptors in the brain. It occurred to us at Fair Oaks that we might be able to give coke addicts who were going through early withdrawal something to keep their dopamine system activated in the absence of cocaine, which would help them to not drop out of treatment.

In the early eighties my colleague Charles Dackis and I conducted some pioneering studies on cocaine addicts. In the first, we gave two patients doses of either bromocriptine or placebo (a look-alike but harmless pill) and asked them to rate the intensity of their cravings on a scale of 0 to 100. During six trials the patients could always tell when they had been given the active drug; their craving ratings fell significantly, from a high of about 80 to a low of about 20. Later we repeated the experiment with 13 patients. Again, we asked them to indicate how severe their cravings were at different points during the day. Then, to intensify their cravings, we asked them to handle a white powder that looked like cocaine (harmless old lactose, a milk sugar) and drug paraphernalia (syringes, pipes, mirrors, and razor blades) to reenact the process of using the drug. They did this for 15 minutes. Then we gave some of the patients bromocriptine, and the rest placebo. The next day we repeated the procedure, but switched the groups: Those that had the drug the first day were given placebo, and vice versa. The patients were then asked to rate the severity of their cravings for the rest of the afternoon.

Bingo! Those who had been given bromocriptine noticed significant declines in their cravings. Eleven of the 13 patients correctly guessed which day they had had the drug. Since these early experiments, the results of which have been generally confirmed by other researchers, bromocriptine has been used with hundreds of recovering coke addicts. The fact that the drug helps snuff out their cravings has made it possible for many of them to stay in treatment and kick their habits entirely.

Bromocriptine works initially as an antidepressant, alleviating the low mood that accompanies the cocaine crash. It also corrects cocaine-induced disturbances in sexual hormones, specifically prolactin, which governs fertility and the secretion of breast milk in women and impotence in men. Studies show that bromocriptine rapidly returns the levels of this hormone to normal and is effective in treating cocaine abusers with sexual dysfunction.

A number of groups are currently doing work to find out if bromocriptine also blocks the euphoric effects of cocaine. If so, treatment with bromocriptine would take care of the two main problems that reinforce cocaine addiction: euphoria and craving. In the future we may be able to develop a strategy for treatment, perhaps using a long-lasting injectable form of a new drug that will help patients by preventing them from getting high off of coke while it wipes out their cravings for the drug.

We are also keeping our eye on other drugs to see if they may play a role in treating cocaine users. Researchers report that other drugs effective against Parkinson's can also decrease cravings, and that a dopamine-acting antidepressant, such as Wellbutrin (bupropion) may help. In addition, Frank Gawin and others have suggested that antidepressants such as nortriptyline or desipramine can help with relapse and alleviate low mood caused by coke use. However, early reports of desipramine's effectiveness have been tempered by Marian Fischman's NIDA Research Center data that shows only a slight beneficial effect with an increased risk of cardiotoxicity, irritability, and anger.

So far I've been describing treatments specifically aimed at the problem of cocaine cravings and at reducing the relapse rates among addicts. One additional problem we have not been able to solve—yet—is cocaine overdose.

During my work with President Reagan's White House Conference for a Drug Free America, we crisscrossed the country meeting with physicians and drug treatment specialists in many communities. We talked about the exciting ways, both actual and promising, of helping addicts overcome their drug slavery. But when it came time to discuss cocaine overdose, the conversation often lapsed into a painful silence.

To illustrate, let me remind you of the story of Len Bias, a healthy young athlete who gambled with cocaine and lost. He was taken to an emergency room where doctors did all they could but in the end watched helplessly as he died. The truth is, Len would have been better off overdosing on heroin.

There's a treatment available for heroin overdose; not so with cocaine. Someday when we have more information about cocaine's receptor in the brain, it should be possible to develop a medication that blocks the acute effects of cocaine, thereby greatly improving our treatment for cocaine overdose. Unfortunately, cocaine toxicity and overdose are still major problems without medical solutions.

There are some strategies that may help relieve a few of the symptoms, however. People experiencing cocaine overdose may suffer hyperthermia—an enormous rise in body temperature. There are reports of patients going from 101 degrees Fahrenheit to 106 in the time it took to use the thermometer. In such cases it may be beneficial—even lifesaving—to dip the person's body in ice water. Patients suffering panic attacks may benefit from antianxiety medications such as Valium (diazepam). Diazepam, or barbiturates such as pentobarbital (Nembutal), may help control cocaine-induced seizures, while other drugs may help alleviate irregular heartbeats or high blood pressure. But symptomatic treatment is not the answer; we need an emergency antidote like naloxone and a long-term blocker like naltrexone.

Given the rising use of crack, and its awesomely addictive powers, a fast-acting treatment to be available nationwide in emergency rooms and ambulances for the entire cocaine overdose syndrome—the most critically severe and least researched problem caused by this drug—ranks high on my wish list. Also, additional research on cocaine receptors in the brain and on the mechanism of cocaine withdrawal remains equally important.

Medical Treatment of Alcoholism

The best approach to treating alcohol abuse is total abstinence, coupled with the support of family, friends, self-help groups such as AA, and outpatient treatment centers when necessary. However, some physicians prescribe a medication called

Antabuse (disulfiram) to help alcoholics in recovery. Antabuse causes any person who drinks even a small amount of alcohol to become violently ill with nausea and vomiting. Antabuse may appear to be the "magic pill" for alcoholism, but in reality it does nothing to address the long-term problems of alcoholics. At best, Antabuse should be used under a doctor's supervision merely as a temporary aid during the first weeks of sobriety, when the risk of relapse is highest. Eventually the alcoholic will learn that the power to resist alcohol comes, not from a pill, but instead partly from within and partly from relying on others for help.

Perhaps in the future medical researchers will discover new medications that will help alcoholics in their struggle. Interestingly, a current medication, naltrexone, used in treating heroin relapse (see below), may someday be used for alcoholism. For now, however, the best strategy for this form of chemical dependency is one involving no chemicals at all.

Medical Treatment of Marijuana Abuse

I can make this short: There's nothing available. Like alcoholism, the way to manage marijuana addiction is with detoxification followed by lifelong abstinence.

Medical Treatment of Heroin Withdrawal

This is one area where medical science can claim some astounding victories.

Elsewhere I've described the role of methadone in managing people addicted to heroin. Briefly, the concept is to replace heroin with methadone, then gradually withdraw the patient from drugs entirely. Sometimes this works, sometimes it doesn't.

Opiate drugs, including methadone, attach themselves to specific receptors in the brain, elbowing the body's own natural painkillers out of their way like shoppers fighting over a K mart blue-light special. Eventually the body gives up the fight and loses its ability to generate its own supply of these natural opiates. Hence, addiction—the user must continually inject a new supply to ward off the pain of withdrawal.

As a medical student at the University of Florida I studied opiate withdrawal in rodents. Along with Steve Zornetzer, I tried to reverse withdrawal by giving a drug that depleted the brain of norepinephrine. With these interests, my teachers at Florida advised me to go to Yale. There, exciting studies were already in progress and dealt with everything from studying single brain cells to anxiety in human and nonhuman primates.

While at Yale, I studied a key site of opiate activity in the brain called the locus coeruleus. With Gene Redmond's and George Aghajanian's ongoing work with rodents as a foundation, we conducted other studies that suggested that without adequate supplies of opiates (natural or otherwise) to regulate this active mass of nerves, the cells there fire wildly and send off a barrage of electrical signals that create a lot of uncomfortable feelings throughout the body. These feelings are the symptoms of withdrawal.

Aghajanian taught me that a drug called clonidine (sold as Catapres), used to treat high blood pressure, works in part by interfering with the activity of cells in the locus coeruleus. In other words, it inhibits their firing and calms things down. Importantly, however, while clonidine is not an opiate drug and will not attach itself to opiate receptors, it does have many opiate-like properties: It relieves pain, causes the pupils to contract, lowers blood pressure, relieves anxiety, slows breathing rate, and produces a degree of sedation.

Back in the mid-1970s, it occurred to me that this inhibitory effect of clonidine might be useful in ridding heroin addicts of their withdrawal symptoms, and make it easier for them to kick their habit. Kleber agreed. Studies on animals and on humans confirmed this effect. It's a source of pride to me that my work with doctors Kleber, Redmond, and Aghajanian at Yale University led to the development of clonidine, the first nonopiate treatment for opiate withdrawal. In the 15 years since this discovery, clonidine has helped thousands of patients get rid of the monkey on their backs. It's a fine example of basic research applied to an age-old problem.

Essentially, clonidine "fools" the brain into thinking it's not suffering from withdrawal when in fact it is. Use of this medication means a person who has been addicted to heroin or maintained on methadone can be *drug-free in less than two weeks.* Released from the prison of withdrawal symptoms, patients can then begin the other aspects of treatment, such as learning how to end their drug-seeking behavior, avoid relapse, and maintain the drug-free state.

A pretty tough challenge.

Enter naltrexone. (Another wonder drug waiting for someone to get it approved and manufactured. Again, we were pioneers.) Like a partner in a tag-team wrestling match, naltrexone, sold under the brand name Trexan, steps in to finish the job that clonidine has started. This drug works by linking up with the opiate landing sites in the brain, thus preventing any other opiates from settling there. A person maintained on naltrexone might shoot up with heroin, but it'd be a waste of time and money; the heroin has nowhere to go—all the parking spots are filled—and so it passes harmlessly out of the body. Naltrexone insures the addict against relapse and overdose. What's more, naltrexone is safe, nonaddicting, long lasting, and produces no euphoria on its own. We clearly showed clonidine's and naltrexone's success in treating patients—especially those patients whose employment status and social supports augmented our medical treatments.

We usually give patients naltrexone orally three times a week. Because it lasts so long in the body before breaking down, naltrexone helps addicts suppress, and eventually overcome, their continuing (but now-weakening) impulse to use drugs.

We've found that when we tell our patients they are taking naltrexone, a drug that completely blocks the effects of heroin, they experience a sense of relief. They realize that they no longer have to struggle with their desire for opiates, and that reduces their anxiety, tension, and depression. They know that, even if they slip, they aren't in danger of complete relapse. In our experience, the only failures we've had in using the one-two punch of clonidine and naltrexone for long-term maintenance are cases where the patients failed to take their medication on schedule. These failures were not due to some flaw in the medications themselves.

I must add, however, that medications alone won't solve all of the problems addicts recovering from opiate use will face. No pill will get them their job back, or repair the damage caused to their relationships with family and friends. In addition to medical treatment, addicts need access to other types of therapy as well, including group, individual, and family therapy. A Twelve Step program such as Narcotics Anonymous can work wonders. More on that in the next part of this book.

In the coming years we will continue to fine-tune our strategy for helping addicts overcome opiates. For example, a medication called lofexidine has many of the same properties as clonidine but without its sedating side effects. In some of our patients on lofexidine, we've seen dramatic relief from anxiety and distress. This drug thus may be more appropriate for some patients, especially those who are being treated as outpatients. We are also exploring the advantages of using a whole spectrum of other medications to manage other aspects of the problem: antidepressants, antihypertensives, and antispasticity drugs, for example. As the billboards say, watch this space for further developments.

Narcotic Antagonists Until recently, any heroin addict trying to quit had two choices: either stop immediately ("cold turkey") or undergo gradual detoxification with methadone. Either choice was loaded with potential problems: the painfully intense cravings of cold turkey versus the difficult and prolonged detoxification with methadone. In either case, the medical community could offer little more than support to recovering addicts.

However, the advent of *naltrexone* gave addicts a medical

alternative to help them through the difficult periods of recovery. Naltrexone is a narcotic antagonist that works by binding itself to opiate receptors in the brain and blocking the effects of opiates. An addict could take copious amounts of heroin and it would have no effect.

A very similar drug called *naloxone* (brand name Narcan) had been used intravenously by emergency room physicians and paramedics since 1971 to reverse narcotic overdoses that previously would have been fatal. Naltrexone offers two major advantages over naloxone—it can be given orally and its effects can last for days. Hence naltrexone can be used in outpatient treatment programs as an excellent means of helping the addict to overcome the temptations of addiction. Unfortunately, addicts who prematurely drop out of the treatment will soon find their temptation returning.

I must stress here that even with the advent of clonidine, Narcan, and naltrexone, the number of heroin addicts has remained relatively stable over the years. This point clearly illustrates that no medical treatment, no matter how effective, can solve the problem of drugs. Still, the search for effective medical treatments continues.

Interestingly, some treatment specialists report having success using a variety of nonmedicinal strategies. Acupuncture—the ancient Chinese art of sticking needles into the skin at certain precise locations—is one such approach. Apparently, for some people at least, the use of needles in the earlobes seems to lessen the symptoms of withdrawal, though heaven only knows why. Perhaps doing so stimulates certain nerves, which in turn stimulate the production of endorphins. Perhaps, too, for addicts in pain, just having someone pay attention to their problem in a caring way may have some effect. A doctor in Hong Kong developed a modern-day version of acupuncture using electrified needles; he reports success in helping his patients lose their desire for heroin.

These exotic treatment methods may hold some promise. At this point, however, we lack the detailed and controlled studies we need to determine exactly how to use them and the patients for whom they may be best suited.

Other Promising Strategies

All people with substance abuse problems are unique. Their physiologies, their genetic and cultural backgrounds, their environment, even the way they think—everything has an impact on their decision to use drugs, on their choice of drug to abuse, and on the way the drug affects their bodies and minds. To serve our patients best, we physicians must use all the tools available to evaluate the problem and choose the method of treatment best suited for each particular individual.

As a biopsychiatrist, I have long urged my colleagues in the mental health field to take advantage of the vast array of laboratory tests and diagnostic imaging devices that exist today to help the treatment-resistant patient. Too often we psychiatrists seem to forget that a patient's mental problems may have a physical basis, and that we as physicians can—indeed must—use every resource to get to the bottom of those problems. Only then will we know which therapy has the best chance of succeeding.

Efforts by Dr. Charles Schuster and the agency he directs, the National Institute on Drug Abuse (NIDA), have been essential in forging the link between science and the treatment of substance abuse. In 1990, NIDA established a research and development program specifically designed to develop new medications for the treatment of drug abuse.

Someday it may be possible to actually create a vaccine against cocaine. This idea is based upon the discovery that cocaine stimulates the user's body to produce anticocaine antibodies.

Within the last decade we've made tremendous strides in our ability to peer inside the living body and watch it work. The CAT (computerized axial tomography) scanner and MRI (magnetic resonance imaging) technique have revealed physical abnormalities that identify alcoholic patients. Even more advanced methods, such as positron emission tomography (PET) scans and other images that show electrical and magnetic activity, also show promise in helping us understand the biological basis of addiction. The PET scanner, for example, lets us watch as drugs migrate through the body, attach to receptor sites, and trigger the release and metabolism of various neurotransmitters. Recently neurologists have devised a magnetic probe that measures muscle function painlessly and without surgery. Such technologies have already proved themselves to be as important to medicine as the X ray was at the beginning of this century.

As one observer wrote, devices that reveal how drugs work in the living body at the molecular and cellular level have given us a "fast track" between the medical researcher's bench and the clinical bedside. Our increasing understanding of the interplay between chemicals and the pathways they take in the brain and body will yield enormous payoffs—not just in the treatment of substance abusers but for everyone.

Good news? *Fabulous* news.

CHAPTER FOURTEEN

Outpatient Treatment

Frankly, I'd rather not have you, or anyone else for that matter, as my hospital's patient.

Does that surprise you? Let me explain.

The ideal place for treating people with drug problems is outside the hospital. Yes, in-hospital treatment works—it works very well. But now, in nine out of ten cases, outpatient care would be my first choice for helping a substance abuser. In fact, at Fair Oaks, we've established Outpatient Recovery Centers (ORC) that have helped thousands of people recover from addiction without the need for hospitalization.

Outpatient treatment can work just as well as hospitalization. It costs less. And many people accept outpatient treatment more willingly, since it carries less of a social stigma. There may simply be more slots available to outpatients, too. Outpatient care is certainly less disruptive to the drug abuser's life; often people can still hold down their jobs and go about most of their daily activities while in therapy. At ORC, we've tailored several different programs to meet the needs of individuals who can still work or attend school while participating in a formal recovery program.

The most important reason, though, is that *in every case of substance abuse, outpatient care will be needed—at some time and to some degree.* It might occur as the first step in the process. Ideally, it will be the only such step. If it fails—a real possibility—then the addict will need to enter a hospital program. But the goal of inpatient care is to return people to a normal life, and by definition there can be no "normal" life inside the hospital. Patients must return to the real world at some point. When they get out, they will need a lot of additional support and follow-up care if they hope to remain drug-free for the rest of their lives.

Most treatment programs in this country fall into one of five categories. I'll discuss the first three types in this chapter.

Outpatient clinics provide counseling and support for people trying to kick their habits while they continue to live and function within the community.

Methadone maintenance programs are aimed specifically at helping heroin addicts get away from needles, leave behind drug-searching behaviors, get a job, and make the transition to a drug-free state.

Residential therapeutic communities are highly structured programs lasting up to 18 months in which addicts live together while working to change the deep-rooted habits and attitudes that contribute to their drug problems.

Detoxification programs are those in which patients stay in a care facility for a few days with the specific goal of "drying out"—ridding their body of drugs.

Chemical dependency programs are usually private inpatient units in hospitals or other facilities where treatment lasts up to four weeks and which offer patients a range of other supportive therapies in addition to detoxification. In the next chapter I will focus on these two types of hospital-based, medically oriented programs.

Characteristics of a Model Outpatient Program

- Advocates total abstinence from all mood-altering drugs.
- Presents accurate and current information about the health hazards of drug use.
- Encourages the patient to change but doesn't resort to lectures or harangues.
- Addresses the patient's age, interests, and special needs.
- Involves parents, spouses, or other important people.
- Emphasizes the present impact of drug use and holds patients accountable for their actions.
- Uses urine testing to assure and monitor compliance.

(Adapted with permission from Mark S. Gold et al. "New Treatments for Opiate and Cocaine Users." *Psychiatric Annals,* April 1986.)

Criteria for Outpatient Care

What should you look for in an outpatient treatment program, either for yourself or someone you care about? There are two main ingredients: sound philosophy and solid structure (see Box above).

As for philosophy, you should make sure that the program advocates *complete abstinence from all drugs.* Permitting "occasional" drug use is both unrealistic and dangerous. Drugs affect the body and the mind; that's why people take them. Trying to get through to people who are pumped full of chemicals is like trying to broadcast television signals to people who have turned off their sets. Addicts in therapy must stay away from all nonprescription drugs if they want to tune in to the message.

The treatment program must also advocate *regular drug testing.* Ideally, urine samples should be collected two or three times a week. Rather than waste time asking the patient questions about drug use and trying to discern whether he is telling the truth, why not have the urine tests provide the answer? Far from being invasive, such testing actually works to build trust between the patient and the caregiver. Even better, it eliminates the denial and self-deceit that so often sabotage treatment. And knowing they have to pass the "whiz quiz" actually helps make patients more able to control their drug urges.

In conjunction with drug testing, the program must clearly spell out the *consequences of failure.* Among the possibilities: temporary suspension from the program; more frequent therapy sessions; more intensive education; or admission (in some cases, readmission) to a hospital.

As for structure, the best programs recognize the different (and, to a degree, overlapping) phases of addiction and recovery, and will offer support at each of these steps along the road to recovery.

The first phase, as I've indicated, is abstinence. For the first 30 to 60 days of treatment, work focuses on making patients drug-free and keeping them that way for at least a month. This goal is both realistic and achievable. To insure compliance, however, the patient should see the therapist every day during this phase to get counseling, support, and education. Together they will explore the patient's reasons for resisting the need to give up drugs. When the user can admit he has a problem and expresses a desire to change, the time is right for the patient to join a peer recovery group.

Another key goal during this first phase is to help people identify the things that trigger their drug urges and work out ways to control—and eventually eliminate—cravings

Addicts need to learn that drug use is largely a conditioned response. One person might discover that he reflexively lights up a joint to defend against the first feelings of boredom. Another person might only turn to crack when she feels the pressure to perform on the job. Many users develop a drug ritual—even as simple as drawing the blinds and lowering the lights. So powerful can such a ritual be that whenever the user enters a room with the blinds drawn, he starts to feel a craving.

A good treatment program recognizes the power of these stimuli, warns patients about them, and teaches techniques for controlling them. (Open the blinds, for example!) One strategy is to conjure up mental pictures of the situations and events that trigger drug use, then imagine and rehearse ways of resisting that temptation. In a sense, this is the "adult" version of the resistance skills techniques taught in schools, as we saw in Chapter Ten. Another method is to have patients draw up lists of alternative steps they can quickly take—everything from a cold shower to calling a trusted friend—to thwart their cravings.

At some point, gradually and under supervision, patients have to reenter the real world. They have to return to settings where triggers exist and do so without succumbing to drug urges. To make it through this phase, patients need long-term support and peer-group therapy.

One study showed that inpatient treatment in a sterile hospital environment was only successful about half as often as outpatient treatment alone. The main difference was that outpatient care helped patients deal directly with these day-to-day challenges of resisting their urges to use drugs.

Many patients refuse to enter treatment because they feel their cravings will always be too strong to resist. That's a myth. Cravings can be managed if the treatment program follows the steps I've just outlined. Remember, a craving need not be acted upon!

As my colleague James Cocores, medical director of the Outpatient Recovery Centers of Fair Oaks, has shown, once addicts have learned to abstain from drugs and control their cravings, the focus of treatment shifts. The emphasis during this second phase is now on anticipating and preventing relapse. To reach this goal and make the necessary changes in life-style, patients need education and support. The danger of relapse has to be acknowledged and confronted. As AA taught us, recovery for a substance abuser is a lifelong process. A treatment program that promises total and absolute freedom from drugs—forever and ever amen—is selling snake oil. Denying the threat of relapse means the program has no policy for dealing with it when it erupts.

The best programs are the ones that recognize the problem of relapse and work actively to avoid it. They know patients are at constant risk of slipping. They realize, too, that once the slip occurs, patients will inevitably suffer a disabling cycle of intense feelings of failure, guilt, and self-loathing. The patient thinks, "Well, I've blown it. I've smoked a joint. Two months of treatment, out the window. I'm already a failure—might as well go the whole nine yards. Where's my crack pipe?"

It's better, of course, if the program teaches the patient to handle the problem more positively. Ideally, the patient's thoughts would run something like this: "Well, there's that slip they warned me about—right on schedule, too. I guess the pressure at work got to be too much for me. Thank goodness I know one slip isn't fatal. I'll call my counselor or go to another meeting. I'll talk about this and ask how I can cope with the pressure better."

Some of the techniques for preventing relapse include: predicting which situations are more likely to trigger cravings; rehearsing strategies for avoiding those situations or for responding to them without resorting to drugs; altering life-style —changing jobs, for example, if necessary; developing drug-free support networks; reinforcing the negative aspects and painful memories of drug use; and working to reduce or cope with stress.

The final phase, which I call consolidation, arrives usually a year or so after treatment begins and continues indefinitely afterwards. By this point patients have learned which strategies work for them and which don't. Often they then graduate to therapy groups that have a different focus. Before, the emphasis was on the day-to-day struggle against drugs; now it's on the long-term aspects of a drug-free life. One goal, for example, is to combat overconfidence, a feeling that often emerges after a patient has managed to avoid drugs for a few months. Also, people who quit using drugs may need help coping with the psychological problems that may emerge once their drug-induced fog has lifted.

Outpatient therapy for drug addiction, like any medical prescription, has to be chosen carefully to address each individual's problems. Mary might need to repair the damage her drug use did to her marriage, while Mike might need to work on improving his relationship with his parents. In addition to individual counseling and peer group therapy, patients may need some combination of family therapy, couples therapy, or vocation rehabilitation. The people who are important in a patient's life need to learn what roles they should play in recovery. They may need to be taught, for example, to withhold money from the patient or to avoid acting as enablers for the patient's destructive behavior. The younger the patient, the more important it is that the entire family become involved in treatment. For more on this, see Chapter Sixteen.

It's a good idea to find a program that focuses on the particular chemical that's being abused. Patients addicted to cocaine, for example, report having much better success if they enter a recovery group that addresses the specific issues related to cocaine and crack addiction. When everyone in a group can identify with a member's suffering, feelings of isolation and loneliness quickly disappear, making the road to recovery that much shorter.

A supermarket gives you a better chance of finding everything on your grocery list than a store that only sells cheese. The same principle applies to drug treatment: Prepackaged, single-product, we-cure-anybody programs are bound to fail. Studies show that patients can benefit more *if* they enter a treatment program that offers a variety of therapies, rather than a program that takes a one-size-fits-all approach.

How can you judge whether a program is good? That's a tough one. High on my wish list for the near future is a set of standards by which we can measure the effectiveness of outpatient treatment methods. One of Herbert Kleber's goals as deputy director for Demand Reduction in the Office of National Drug Control Policy is to evaluate treatment programs and approaches. We need a kind of "consumer's report," or scorecard, showing which plans work best. To generate such a report, we need objective standards.

One obvious measure is the relapse rate after a certain period of time among graduates of a given program. Ideally, in our market economy, only those programs with the highest success rates (and thus the lowest relapse rates) would qualify for government funds and patient referrals, and would thus remain in operation. Those programs whose patients proved able to resume working and continue working or not be highly prone to relapse would stay in business.

Other ways of measuring success include drop-out rates, arrest records, employment history, attendance at school, participation in self-help groups, or results of drug tests. For the most part, this data is short term. To be fair, such report cards also need to factor in the differences between treatment programs, including length of treatment, patients' individual histories of drug use and treatment, extent of mental or physical illness, employment and education, criminal record, and family relationships.

Group Therapy

We humans are social animals. Like bees and ants, we depend on each other for survival. Everybody—whether a drug addict or not—needs to be connected to a strong, thriving peer group. For any one of us, developing such a support network is important; for a drug user especially, belonging to a group can literally be a matter of life and death.

A good outpatient treatment program is one that first works to help the patient become abstinent and drug-free. At some point in that process patients will be ready to benefit from self-help groups like AA or NA and a structured, medically supervised group therapy. Ideally, this group should be run by a team made up of a medical professional and a recovering addict who has been clean for several years. The group should meet many times a week as part of a broader program that includes family, individual, or other types of therapy as needed.

In group sessions, addicts get the chance to express their

feelings about their drug urges and the way drugs have affected their thinking. They can trade ideas on ways to avoid relapse. In group therapy, patients learn that others share their problems and that they are not alone in their struggle. In the process they realize that it's possible to develop and adopt an entirely new belief system, one that isn't founded on the use of drugs.

Elsewhere in this book I've described how cocaine depletes the brain's supply of the neurotransmitter dopamine. Once I was asked whether group therapy, or any kind of talk therapy for that matter, works because it produces emotional responses that in turn stimulate dopamine synthesis. My first reaction was no, of course not. Then it dawned on me that, well, there may be something to that idea. We neurobiologists are highly aware of the connection between our emotions and our physical well-being. Certainly it doesn't tax the imagination to imagine patients feeling so elated by their experience in group sessions that the neurotransmitter channels are kicked into higher gear. So in a sense, yes, taking part in group sessions may indeed directly counteract the physical problems caused by the use of drugs, especially cocaine.

Ideally, the insights gained in group sessions become the raw material for further processing when the patient meets with the doctor for individual sessions. In private sessions, where the patient gets the caregiver's full attention, the conversation can focus more intensely on the patient's relationships, sexuality, self-esteem, and problems with the family. You can see, I hope, how all forms of therapy complement and enhance each other.

Role of Twelve Step (Self-Help) Groups

At some point in the process, the patient will be ready to move on to a different kind of group, such as a self-help group that is not run by a medical professional, while continuing individual therapy as necessary with a doctor.

For many years drug treatment specialists belonged to one

of two camps. In one camp were those who believed that only a classic by-the-numbers psychiatric approach would work. They used psychotherapy to uncover the hidden reasons a person felt compelled to abuse drugs or alcohol. This strategy works for some.

In the other camp were people who saw psychiatrists as the enemy of the addict and who thus believed in a purely nonmedical strategy. The Twelve Step approach developed by Alcoholics Anonymous was often seen as representing this point of view. To say that "AA opposes medicine" risks stereotyping that philosophy. Nonetheless, there is a grain of truth in the stereotype. There was, and from some quarters there still may be, hostility directed at psychiatrists from the Twelve Step camp. Some of these AA-type groups promote total abstinence from addictive substances but forget that there are people who do indeed have psychiatric problems, problems that may be completely unrelated to drug use but which make the addiction worse and which will respond to psychiatric care.

The good news is that these two camps are moving closer. In recent years the psychiatric profession has acknowledged that, to be successful, treatment *must* offer group therapy. They realize a Twelve Step group is one very powerful way to help their patients meet other people who deeply understand their agony. Group sessions—whether offered by Twelve Step programs or through other volunteer or private agencies—offer positive role models, a ready-made support network, and a forum for solving problems.

And Twelve Step programs have moved forward, too. Modern groups realize that many substance abusers do indeed have other psychiatric problems. Such groups now recognize they are of most value to their members when they help them get all the kinds of care, including medical care, that they need.

The phrase "Twelve Step" refers to the fact that other groups—Cocaine Anonymous, Narcotics Anonymous, Overeaters Anonymous—have adopted the famous AA approach in order to address other forms of dependency. Each of these free programs is run completely by volunteers who are themselves recovering substance abusers. I distinguish between self-help groups such as Twelve Step programs and other types of group therapy, some of which may be run entirely by trained professionals and which may or may not charge members for the service.

As I've made clear elsewhere in this book, any medical drug treatment plan that doesn't include group therapy is not doing everything possible. In groups, older members offer newer ones the benefit of their experience. Groups also focus on issues of great interest to each member, and are a great way to share new information quickly and with the urgency of personal concern. Members share "war stories" and explain their ways of surviving in the real world. Hearing such stories helps shyer members open up and share some of their own experiences. For an addict overwhelmed with shame, seeing so many other people in the same boat can be a tremendous relief. Membership motivates people to stay drug-free, but lets them see that loving arms await to catch them should they slip.

Members of Twelve Step groups admit, to themselves and publicly, that they cannot drink or use drugs. In doing so they give up their illusion that they have control over their substance abuse. They replace that illusion with the reality—reinforced just by taking part in group sessions—that they are working to achieve self-mastery over their behavior. As Edward K. Rynearson wrote in *Psychiatric Annals:* "Recovered addicts and supportive family members and friends can offer a more immediate and relevant social matrix for reinforcement and recovery than psychiatry can alone."

Though anyone may benefit from a Twelve Step approach, there's evidence that suggests certain groups respond especially well. Adolescent marijuana users, for example, may ignore adult guidance but will often respond to help from someone their own age. In groups, positive behavior is reinforced, while negative behaviors and attitudes are identified and discouraged. Women benefit from groups because such programs provide structure and clear guidance for behavior and help reinforce the member's sense of identity.

There's one other group of people who need special attention: the substance abusers who have some other form of psychiatric illness. These dual-diagnosis patients need programs that address both aspects of their condition. Often, for example, alcoholics who are also clinically depressed join AA and get sober but, because of their depression, they don't notice the same improvement in their lives that they see in the lives of other members. They may interpret the lack of change as a failure on their part, which only increases their risk of slipping. If the person can't shake the depression, others in the group may accuse the member of self-pity.

The flip side of the problem is the patient who attends AA and also gets treatment from a psychiatrist for depression. There's a tendency, understandable perhaps, for others in the self-help group to blame doctors or the treatment they prescribe for causing, or worsening, the depression.

Some patients have mental illnesses that make it hard for them to attend, and thus benefit from, Twelve Step groups. People who are anxious, paranoid, or who have certain phobias —for example, fear of leaving the house or fear of germs or contamination—may not make it to the meeting room. However, there are some psychiatric disorders that do respond well to group involvement. According to Harvard University researchers Drs. Roger D. Weiss and Steven M. Mirin, many patients with mood disorders thrive in a structured peer-support program with a hopeful message and clear guidelines for action. Patients with borderline personality disorders like having unambiguous rules ("don't drink, go to meetings, ask for help"). They also like knowing that meetings are held regularly and dependably, and that they have access to a large group of people who willingly offer their support.

Part of the good news, as I mentioned, is that the old animosity between psychiatrists and self-help groups is being replaced by mutual respect and cooperation. Another part is that self-help groups such as one called Double Trouble now exist that are designed specifically for patients with a dual diagnosis.

Residential Treatment

In a sense residential treatment programs are both "fish and fowl." They are inpatient programs in the sense that addicts agree to live with others in a therapeutic community for extended lengths of time—up to two years. But not all of them are run by doctors and they are thus not necessarily medical programs; they focus instead on helping patients learn, day by day, how to take responsibility for their own lives and for the lives of others within that community. In that sense, they are outpatient programs—therapy groups that live together 24 hours a day, using behavioral and cognitive methods to change their actions and attitudes.

Two of the best-known residential programs are Phoenix House and Daytop Village. In an article in *The New York Times,* Michel Marriott described a Phoenix House treatment center located in the Bronx as "sanity and order amid anarchy." This particular house is a five-story apartment building. Inside, the members lead highly regimented lives—they know in advance when they will eat, study, sleep, and awaken. Men must be clean shaven; no one, including women, may wear jewelry. Residents report that the strict dress code, sometimes calling for ties and jackets, helps build a better sense of self-image. The philosophy of Phoenix House—a phoenix was a mythological bird that arose from its own ashes—is to break addicts of their past habits and build up new, more positive identities.

The program at Phoenix House lasts at least 18 months, although many residents don't manage to stay that long. They begin the program by working at menial tasks—sweeping, washing floors, cleaning bathrooms. Eventually they earn the right to take on more responsibility. At the same time they undergo intensive counseling to help them resist drugs. If they break any of the strict rules (no use of drugs; no sexual contact among members; keep sleeping quarters clean and tidy; and so on) they lose privileges, such as weekend leaves, and may be demoted from the favored jobs they had worked so hard to earn. There is no real privacy, but residents may not enter each other's rooms without an invitation.

Residents participate in rap sessions, job-training seminars, and classes to prepare them for the graduate equivalency diplomas. Group sessions are the cornerstone of the program. During some sessions they may write and perform inspirational songs or skits. On weekends, things relax somewhat; there may be videos to watch or supervised trips off the premises.

Phoenix House was founded by former heroin addicts in 1967. Today there are six treatment centers in New York and four in California serving addicts, who can be as young as 14 but who are mostly between 20 and 40. The program is paid for by contributions and by the members' public assistance checks. Phoenix House has also developed drug education curriculums for use in schools.

Residents who slip and return to drugs are dealt with severely. According to *The New York Times,* one member had to sit at a table in a hallway and talk for days to fellow residents, one at a time, about his actions. The program is a relative bargain, at $15,000 a year, and the dropout rate is as high as 50 to 60 percent. However, those who do make it have a very good shot at remaining drug-free. According to Dr. Mitchell S. Rosenthal, president of the Phoenix House Foundation, only 5 percent of the graduates from one residential group and one percent from another had relapsed five years after leaving the program.

Another residential program is Daytop Village. Founded in the mid-1960s and still run by Monsignor William O'Brien, Daytop has grown from a house on Staten Island to an international movement with rehabilitation centers all over the United States and Canada, as well as Italy, Spain, Thailand, Ireland, Brazil, Malaysia, Israel, Sweden, Germany, and the Philippines. Except for Alcoholics Anonymous, Daytop is the largest drug treatment program in the world.

In Daytop's facility in the Catskill Mountains, for example, nearly 200 drug addicts live and work together for up to two years. According to its founder, Daytop doesn't go along with the notion that addiction is a biological problem; rather, they see drug use as a symptom of family problems. The monsignor describes Daytop as a "family-repair station."

New members begin their residency by undergoing a barrage of constant stimulation and suggestions about their drug problems. As in Daytop's forerunner, the Synanon treatment community, older members work on newer ones by humiliating them and calling them names. Some observers call this "brainwashing." Whatever the label, it seems to work. Once the member's will has been broken, the older residents switch to the technique of "love-bombing," showering their new member with love and encouragement. Like Phoenix, residents take on menial tasks and earn their way up the ladder. Violations of strict rules are punished harshly, reflecting the philosophy that relapsing into drug use is fraught with danger.

These residential programs can bring about a deep and profound change in some of their members. They can be very effective and meaningful for those who endure them. Obviously I am more proficient in the medically oriented strategy, but I recognize the fact that residential groups, like other forms of treatment, are striving for the same end: the patient's total spiritual transformation. I have seen these programs work wonders, especially for teenagers. If it works for a person, then I am all for it.

Other Issues in Outpatient Treatment

Elsewhere in this book I've explained how methadone is used in helping wean addicts away from heroin. Methadone clinics are a form of outpatient treatment directed exclusively at heroin users, who are registered and thus able to receive free doses of the synthetic opiate. Methadone replaces the extreme craving for heroin and can allow addicts to return to work. Withdrawal from methadone is less troublesome; the goal is to eventually free the user from reliance on any drug at all.

Other patient groups have needs that an outpatient program must address if it is to do any good. For example, as I've explained, many crack addicts are particularly sensitive to the environmental cues that trigger their cravings. Treatment must work long and hard to extinguish those cravings. One of the leaders in our field, Dr. Charles P. O'Brien of the University of Pennsylvania, shows his outpatients videotapes of dealers selling drugs. He provokes craving to teach users that it can be provoked and that it can be controlled or even extinguished. By doing so he gets the message across that just because addicts see a sale taking place doesn't mean they have to succumb to temptation. However, the cravings are so deeply rooted, he says, that even after 50 such sessions some people still feel them.

Women who need outpatient therapy have it especially rough. They may need access to child care, medical care especially aimed at their health problems, or a halfway house. Because so many of them suffer from troubled relationships with the men in their lives, they often benefit from the loving support of an all-women self-help group. Recently President Bush cited as an example of success an outpatient treatment program at Northwestern University in Chicago that focuses on the needs of pregnant addicts. By addressing their special needs, this program manages to keep 40 percent of its patients drug-free and to help 60 percent of them at least reduce their drug use significantly.

Treatment of elderly patients, especially alcoholics, will work best if it takes into account the problems associated with aging. Some elderly patients, victims of years of substance abuse, may need to be guided carefully into a group to help them learn all over again how to interact with other people without resorting to chemicals. Those who are clinically depressed need antidepressant medications, use of which must be carefully managed, as must therapy for any other existing medical problems. They may also need a social worker to help them resolve family issues or other problems, such as coming up with money to pay rent, utility, or food bills.

The Relapse Trap

It may seem strange to you that I mention programs with a 60 percent success rate, or even a 40 percent success rate, and that I do so with pleasure. "What?" you may be thinking. "Less than *half* of the patients lose their addiction? You call that good news?"

Yes I do. So deadly, so powerful is our enemy that for a program to save even one patient is cause for universal celebration. Naturally, I'd be ecstatic if we could cure everybody. But, for many addicts, a cure is only a pipe dream. Alcoholism and drug addiction are chronic, lifelong illnesses prone to relapse. The sad fact that many treatments fail to help patients, no matter how brilliantly that treatment is designed, is one reason I campaign so strongly for prevention. The best, indeed the only, way to cure people of addiction is to prevent them from ever using drugs in the first place.

Thus, I close this chapter with a final nod of adversarial respect for the worst demon I confront as a drug therapist: relapse.

Our awareness of the drive to relapse is a fairly new development. That's part of the good news, that we now have a clear picture of the problem we're trying to solve. As Dr. O'Brien remarked, "Relapse is so common that it's almost inevitable." He adds, "This is treatment. We don't cure anybody."

In Chapter One I mentioned my early work in which I described the phenomenon called the state dependency of memory. Briefly, this means you can only fully recall something that happened or that you learned in a drug state when you are in that same state. In addiction treatment, this principle means that once drug-free, it's extremely difficult for a patient to truly remember what being an addict was like. Sober addicts may remember their behavior, but they can't tap into the emotional memory of their pain and suffering. Thus, patients who slip and use a mood-altering drug, even after years of sobriety, risk opening the dungeon door and freeing all the old monsters they had held at bay: compulsion, loss of will, denial. Addiction never dies; it merely sleeps.

The trick is to teach the patient that a relapse is only prevented one day at a time by active means. As my colleague Dr. Arnold Washton has shown, every relapse or slip is not the same. Relapse may be statistically inevitable but that doesn't mean treatment has failed. At best, relapse is a kind of small earthquake that releases some of the pressure and which may help forestall a bigger one. Relapse helps expose areas where further work is needed—how to manage stress, for example, or where changes in lifestyle must be made.

There is no "antirelapse" pill or shot we can give patients to inoculate them from relapse. Instead, strategies focus on education and on making better use of group support networks.

Before we turn to a discussion of inpatient care, one last point. I believe in the value of a carefully planned outpatient program, one that combines individual therapy, group therapy, self-help strategies, and medical treatment as needed. But I realize that such a program is not the only answer. Treatment programs are, in a sense, nothing more than vehicles; some are cars, some are boats, some are planes. Patients need to be shown how to operate those vehicles. Each one is different, but still each might take patients where they want to go. If it doesn't, we caregivers have to shift our strategy and show our patients how to enter and operate another vehicle, one more suited to their needs and abilities.

Sometimes that shift involves a stay in the hospital, as I'll describe in the next chapter.

CHAPTER FIFTEEN

Inpatient Treatment

We who help people with substance abuse problems have a saying: To observe the success of inpatient treatment, watch the patient's feet. If they stay in one place, everything's fine (for now); if they are moving toward the door, there's trouble.

Getting those feet to stay put is part of the challenge of treatment. As caregivers, our task is to get the good news across to drug users: Their situation is not hopeless. Quite the opposite. Treatment programs turn lives around, giving hope where once there was nothing but despair.

Forty years ago there was only one drug addiction treatment center in the United States. Today there are perhaps 9,000 programs serving just over 600,000 addicts at any given time. In four decades drug treatment has blossomed into a $3-billion-a-year industry. The cost of some of these programs can be quite high; of course, the cost of no treatment is even higher.

Are these programs doing any good? The answer is yes. One key study found that, on average, up to 80 percent of substance abusers treated for three months or longer had reduced their drug use significantly, and that fully 50 percent were still completely drug-free a year after treatment ended.

Cynics reading such statistics will point out that half the users failed to kick their habits entirely. I prefer to see that the glass is half full. As I've indicated, so powerfully addicting are the drugs we are fighting, and so strong is the tendency to relapse, that to save anyone, let alone half of the people who enter treatment, is cause for celebration. And of course some treatment plans have better success rates than others.

The best facilities recognize that addiction is a medical illness and treat it as such. The approach developed at Synanon, a live-in community of narcotic addicts, assumed that drug users had an "addictive personality," and treatment was aimed at breaking this personality down and building up a new one. To my way of thinking, the basic premise is false. The patients' disease—addiction—causes their personalities to become sick, not the other way around.

Treatment begins with intervention, as I described in Chapter Nine. You can't treat someone who isn't there, nor can you wait for an addict to walk up to you and ask for help. The good news is that treatment can begin at any stage of the descent into addiction and still work. Of course, the earlier the intervention, the better the chances. And remember that treatment is, at best, merely the first of many events in the process of recovery. The main goal of treatment is to give addicts the sense of personal responsibility they need to take the further steps necessary for remaining drug-free. As we saw in the previous chapter, still to come is a lifelong, day-to-day struggle against drugs.

Site of Treatment: In the Hospital or Out?

When outpatient care is not possible, or has failed in the past, hospitalization can be a powerful tool for breaking the cycle of addiction. When patients are under around-the-clock care, they can't readily get at the drugs that caused them trouble in the first place. They can also take advantage of the many types of therapy (individual, group, creative, and so on) the hospital offers. A stay in a treatment facility helps by removing patients from the environment—the home, the streets—that may have led to their trouble in the first place. Being in a place where dedicated and caring people are working, literally night and day, to help them overcome their addiction shows them that it is possible to become drug-free and stay that way.

Another plus is that doctors can do full medical and psychiatric evaluations. Such observations reveal whether the patient has any coexisting problems—medical problems or clinical depression, for example—that need additional treatment. Many of these problems only emerge, and can only be properly evaluated, after detoxification and during continuous, 24-hour observation over a period of several drug-free days.

Hospitalization may not be right, or even necessary, for all patients. As we've seen, for many reasons—cost being but one —outpatient treatment is usually preferable. People who are highly motivated to get better, and who have a satisfying job and strong support among family, friends, or other social networks, are best able to benefit from outpatient programs. The same goes if the person doesn't need to be detoxified or is in no immediate medical or psychiatric danger.

However, in my experience, many patients go through a number of unsuccessful attempts to change their habits on their own, without medical help. They come in for treatment when they realize they need help breaking the cycle of drug abuse. Once admitted, they see the value of a locked unit with 24-hour supervision. They also benefit from taking part in hospital peer group discussions and from joining programs that will continue after discharge.

How do we identify those people most likely to benefit from inpatient care? One measure is whether they have tried to get better and failed. Another is whether they vehemently deny having a problem that is obvious to everyone else. Addicts should also be hospitalized if a psychiatric disturbance impairs their judgment or their ability to function, or if there is a risk of suicide or other self-destructive behavior. A person who has

Should a Drug User Be Hospitalized?

1. How severe is the drug abuse problem? Is the drug use so uncontrollable that the user can't stop at all? Is the person using large amounts of drugs—i.e., smoking crack or using IV drugs daily?
2. Is the person physically addicted to several drugs? If so, will he or she need to be detoxified?
3. Are severe psychiatic and behavioral problems present as a result of drug use? Have other medical problems occurred, such as infections of the sinus or liver? Has the person become suicidal or violent?
4. Is the user unable to function on the job, at school, or at home? Can the user take care of himself or herself, go to work, relate to other people?
5. Has the user tried outpatient therapy without success?

(Adapted from Mark S. Gold, M.D. *The Facts About Drugs and Alcohol, Third Revised Edition,* New York: Bantam Books, 1988, p. 122.)

repeated treatment failures or who has medical problems—seizures, cardiac disease, infections—should enter a hospital treatment program. Sometimes people, such as drug dealers, need to be removed from an environment that provides easy access to drugs.

Another indication is the user's choice of drugs. People who are chronic crack smokers or freebasers, or those who use IV drugs or who are addicted to many drugs at the same time, should probably be hospitalized.

If you are wondering whether an inpatient program is right for you or for someone you are concerned about, answer the questions in the Box above.

Some families resist hospitalizing the drug user because they are embarrassed or they fear the stigma that our society, unfortunately, attaches to people who need psychiatric help. But remember: It's easier to endure embarrassment and fear than grief and guilt when a user dies because he didn't get help.

Indications for Inpatient Treatment of Cocaine Dependency

- Chronic freebase, crack, or intravenous use
- Concurrent dependency on other addictive drugs or alcohol
- Serious medical or psychiatric problems
- Severe impairment of psychological functioning
- Insufficient motivation for outpatient treatment
- Lack of family and social supports
- Failure in outpatient treatment

(Reprinted with permission from *Postgraduate Medicine,* McGraw-Hill Health Care Publications.)

Interestingly, people who snort cocaine are less likely to need hospitalization than crack smokers or abusers of other substances. Intranasal users can usually stop taking the drug abruptly without needing to be given substitute drugs for withdrawal. However, hospitalization is called for in severe cases: for example when the desire for cocaine has replaced other basic survival drives, such as the drive for food; when drug use leads to psychosis; or when abstaining from the drugs results in severe problems with one's ability to function. (See Box above.)

One other point: The goal of treatment is to return patients to a normal life. There can be no "normal" life inside the hospital. But while the treatment comes to an end after a few weeks or months, the cravings for drugs, especially cocaine, can persist for years. Any treatment program worth its salt *must* take into account the long-term needs of the patient, including the need to prevent relapse. Without long-term follow-up and ongoing outpatient care, an inpatient program is like the sound of one hand clapping.

Recipe for an Inpatient Treatment Program

All effective treatment plans share key elements in common. Rule number one for any drug treatment program is *total abstinence from all mood-altering chemicals.* Programs that offer psychotherapy while a person continues to use drugs only prolong the addiction.

The next requirement is *careful evaluation of the patient's condition*—physical, mental, social. During the initial interview, the physician learns the history and scope of the problem and its impact on the patient's life. There will follow a physical examination aimed at turning up signs of heart disease, infections, or other side effects of drug use.

Drug users are notorious liars, deniers, and forgetters—some of them are actually surprised if somebody believes them. I would rather buy a car from Joe Isuzu than take an addict's word about the extent of his or her drug history or current problem. An addict's "memory" lapses may be due to denial or to attempts to gain more "medicine" from his doctor. In any case, *laboratory and diagnostic tests* are crucial. These tests give us objective information about the extent of drug use and damage to the body and the brain. They also reveal whether the patient's symptoms may stem from some cause other than drug abuse. Immediately after the interview the physician should collect blood and urine samples—supervised, to prevent cheating—and ship them off for analysis. Such testing must continue throughout the treatment, both to monitor progress and to detect whether the person is somehow still using drugs even though hospitalized.

Testing lets the staff focus on therapy and forget about being policemen or investigators. Treatment must involve the entire family. Thus a *family evaluation* has to be a part of the process. Especially in the case of adolescent substance abusers, parents must take an active role in therapy. Some families tend to believe (or want to believe) that by turning over their child to a doctor's care they absolve themselves of any further responsibility. No so. They must be made aware that without their continuing involvement, both during and after the inpatient program, the child is even likelier to relapse. An evaluation may also uncover the family's underlying attitudes or factual misconceptions that led the children to abuse drugs in the first place. Once spotted, these problems can then be addressed during family therapy sessions.

Evaluation is an ongoing process. After they have been drug-free for a period of days *patients must be reevaluated.* That's the only way we can get a sense of their true moods. We can't just rely on reports from the family. Addicts may have been using drugs for so long—years, in many cases—that no one (including the patient) has any realistic idea what their personalities are like in the drug-free state.

At Fair Oaks, we've found that perhaps half of cocaine addicts, and about 10 percent of alcoholics, meet the criteria for major depression after they have been detoxified. Perhaps 20 percent demonstrate some symptoms of attention-deficit hyperactivity disorder. If we aren't careful—if we don't reevaluate patients to spot these signs of trouble—we won't be able to treat them properly. Failure to manage depression or other psychiatric problems drives many patients back to their drugs.

Detoxification is another critical component. The body is an amazing machine that can break down and eliminate vast quantities of harmful substances. In many cases the only thing needed for detox is time. Of course, when the liver has been damaged, through excess consumption of alcohol, for example, there is danger that poisons will build up and lead to seizures, coma, even death.

All drug treatment programs *must* detoxify patients. Some people whose only treatment is to attend meetings of Alcoholics Anonymous or Narcotics Anonymous fail to kick their habits. One reason is simple: They drop out. Since drugs stimulate their own taking, the user must first flush them from the body so that other aspects of treatment have a chance to work.

We know that alcohol damages the basic structure of the

brain, changing its ability to control thinking and behavior. We used to think such damage was irreversible. But here's some good news hot off the wire: It appears this chemically induced damage may correct itself *if* the patient stops drinking completely. In some people—even those with extensive histories of drinking—total recovery can occur, at least as far as behavior is involved. More good news: The younger the alcoholic, the better the chance that the damaged brain can be repaired. What's the bottom line? Detoxification and abstinence give drug and alcohol abusers their best shot at getting back to normal.

Medical management is often needed. This may mean treating illnesses that result from abuse. Or it may mean using medications to help wean patients from drugs—fighting fire with fire, as it were—and help them stay drug-free. More on that in a moment.

All treatment programs, inpatient or otherwise, must provide *supportive therapy* that meets the patient's needs. Some examples include:

• *Family therapy*—essential for success—improves communications among family members. What's more, it develops self-awareness and insight, not just into the patient's problems but into that of the family's as a whole.

• *Group therapy* helps patients gain perspective through contact with other people in the same boat. In discussions led by a trained counselor, patients work on improving their skills in social interaction, communication, and problem solving.

• *Individual therapy* is aimed at patients who need special attention or who are reluctant to participate in group therapy.

• *Education* is very much a form of therapy, especially in dealing with substance abusers. Learning the facts about drugs dispels myths and overcomes the rationalizations that perpetuate addiction.

• *Behavioral therapy* focuses on changing the habits that inflame the addiction. One method is aversive conditioning, in which the patient learns to associate negative feelings with drug use. Another method is to draw up a contract that spells out the consequences of behavior—for example, having to come back to the hospital if the patient is ever caught with drugs. However, many behavioral strategies fail to remain effective once the patient has left the doctor's immediate supervision.

The last ingredient in the recipe for treatment is *follow-up care* through counseling and continuing access to therapy. It takes incredible stamina and willpower for recovering addicts to remaining drug-free forever; quite understandably, most find it impossible to avoid relapse entirely. Without ongoing support through follow-up care, they may not stand a chance.

Medical Strategies for Treating Specific Addictions

Marijuana Many substance abusers smoke pot, but they don't usually identify that as their reason for seeking treatment. Lately that's changing. Perhaps due to its increased potency, marijuana is cited by more and more addicts as their primary drug of abuse. They are surprised, though, when they find out we know more about treating heroin addiction than we do about treating people hooked on marijuana.

Successful treatment of marijuana addiction, like any addiction therapy, is based on the idea that the patient has a physiological illness, not a personality disorder or a moral failing. Treatment calls for the old one-two punch: detox, followed by lifelong abstinence. There are no medications that can help us win the battle, as there are with, for example, heroin addiction. In some cases, however, it's possible that an antidepressant (such as desipramine) can help patients get over the hump during the withdrawal phase by relieving fatigue, irritability, and depression. Marijuana addiction rarely calls for inpatient care, unless the person has other medical or psychiatric problems, lacks social supports such as family, or is prone to relapse during outpatient treatment.

In any case, treatment is apt to be a long and frustrating process, for patient and doctor alike. The problem is made worse because addicts typically adopt a stance of denial, deception, and hostility. Nonetheless, a good treatment program for marijuana—or any addiction—should include: complete abstinence from all drugs; access to accurate, up-to-date facts; activities geared to the patient's age and background; and involvement of the family. Patients should be held accountable for their behavior, and should not be shielded from the consequences of their actions.

Oh, and one more thing: The program *must* use frequent urine testing.

Other treatment can be aimed at the specific complications of marijuana abuse. For example, patients experiencing panic or "flashbacks" respond well to supportive therapy and reassurance; in severe cases, however, an antianxiety drug may also help. Patients with psychosis—disorganized thinking, paranoia, aggression, and hallucinations—react well to short-term hospitalization and low doses of antipsychotic medications.

Cocaine The first goal of inpatient treatment for cocaine abuse is to break the cycle of compulsive use while providing a safe, structured drug-free environment for recovery. As I described in Chapter Seven, an abstinent coke binger may go through three phases. The first, lasting about four days, begins with agitation, loss of appetite, and acute cravings, followed by fatigue, exhaustion, depression, irritability, nausea, shaking, increased appetite, oversleeping, and loss of craving.

In the second phase, lasting up to ten weeks, the patient notices improvements in mood and sleep, but the cravings persist and are easily triggered. One patient told me he felt a craving for crack whenever he heard the click of a cigarette lighter. The patient is in greatest danger of relapse during this phase.

In the first phase, symptoms fade out over time, but there is persistent danger that cravings will recur. This pattern is predictable in any coke addict, but is usually more severe in crack smokers, freebasers, and IV users, or those who use more than a gram of cocaine per day.

Each of these phases calls for a different treatment strategy. As we saw in Chapter Thirteen, bromocriptine helps during the acute withdrawal phase because it reduces the cravings that often cause outpatients to relapse and inpatients to sign out of the hospital. What's more, bromocriptine helps relieve other symptoms of withdrawal, including depression, irritability, low energy, and disturbed sleep. Side effects may include headache, sedation, lower blood pressure, or nausea, but reports of such effects are rare. I've never seen a patient get "high" from bromocriptine; that's important, since a tranquilizer called Xanax has been known to induce euphoria in some patients, especially alcoholics. Usually we don't have to prescribe bromocriptine for longer than two weeks.

Antidepressants such as desipramine help during the period of persistent depression and long-term withdrawal, but it usually takes several days, even weeks, before the patient may notice their effects. It's best if the antidepressant doesn't cause sedation; patients suffering the post-coke blues are highly sensitive to this side effect.

Many continuous cocaine abusers have a severe nutritional or vitamin deficiency for at least one vitamin. (Not surprising, given that most of them would rather snort, smoke, or shoot up than eat). The brain needs vitamins and proteins to keep its electrochemical signal system working efficiently. Good treatment means paying attention to diet; if we can correct the nutritional imbalances, we take a big step toward restoring the patient's brain to good working order.

Heroin As we saw in Chapter Thirteen, the blood pressure medication clonidine works to relieve the acute symptoms of withdrawal from opiates and helps smooth the process of detoxification. Over a two-week period, clonidine reverses the impact of opiates on thinking, mood, and the body. It's quicker and more effective than detox carried out with methadone. After detoxification, the patient can start taking naltrexone, which blocks the euphoric effects of opiates and thus prevents readdiction.

One other point: Clonidine even helps babies born to heroin-addicted mothers to make it through their first painful week as they suffer through the process of withdrawal.

There are a few drawbacks with the use of clonidine to treat heroin addicts. It's possible, though not likely, that patients may abuse the drug. They may also develop tolerance to it—they get used to the medication and may need higher doses.

Some evidence suggests other medications may one day prove to be useful. Guanfacine and guanabenz, known as alpha-2 agonists because they stimulate a certain part of the nervous system, have some of the same effects as clonidine but last longer and have fewer side effects. Other possibilities include interferon, a protein secreted by the body's cells to fight off infection, and verapamil, an antihypertensive that is sometimes used to treat manic depression.

Though treatment with medications is very effective in breaking addiction, it is just one small part of the overall picture. The person must learn that there is life after detoxification. Therapy must include some combination of counseling, psychotherapy, and participation in a peer support group if the patient is to stay abstinent long enough to recover. At least as important, if not more so, are long-term rehabilitation and therapy to change attitudes, behavior, or environmental factors that may prolong drug use.

Many drugs users come from worlds where they know only poverty, crime, and drugs. Giving them a pill won't make those horrors vanish forever, although many use illicit drugs in a futile attempt to escape for a little while. These people need a host of social services, counseling, and even job training. A treatment plan isn't complete—nor will it work—unless it addresses the patient's need to find a fulfilling life within the community. Family therapy, AA, social case work, and other methods all contribute toward that goal.

The Challenge of the Dual Diagnosis

Some patients suffer not just from drug addiction but from some other psychiatric disorder as well. In order for the patient to be treated properly, both diagnoses must be made.

It's not uncommon, for example, for alcoholics to have a panic or anxiety disorder. If an alcoholic stops drinking and a week later goes into a panic, many people would dismiss the problem, saying "Tsk, tsk, poor old Mac—off the sauce for a few days and already in trouble." What's happening is not that Mac needs a drink; instead, his new sobriety has allowed his underlying panic disorder to emerge. Mac needs to be treated for this condition—imipramine does nicely—or else he may return to drinking, feeling, wrongly, that booze is his only hope. Sure, living without alcohol can cause an alcoholic to feel panicky for a while, but a careful doctor will distinguish between that temporary sense of panic and a coexisting anxiety disorder.

Alcoholics diagnosed as also having bipolar disease—mood swings—often respond well to lithium and perhaps psychotherapy as well. The use of antidepressants for alcoholics with depression is still somewhat controversial. And alcoholics should not be given the tranquilizers known as benzodiazepines, since there is a high possibility that they will begin to abuse these drugs.

As a rule of thumb, patients with a dual diagnosis must be treated for their substance abuse problem *first*. For many patients, especially women, addiction becomes a channel for expressing anger, sadness, or shame. Only when active substance abuse stops can we diagnose these other problems. Patients need to be educated about the two or more different illnesses they have, and must understand that each has to be treated separately and seriously. In most cases, freeing people from their drug slavery results in great improvements, not just in their moods and their personalities, but in their whole outlook on life.

Measuring Results

Treatment works.

But success depends on a lot of factors. If a person's addiction is comparatively mild, or if we catch it early enough, we have a big head start. Another boost comes from strong family support—concerned parents or a loving spouse.

It also helps if the person is highly motivated to get better. Attitude is crucial. Recently, in New Jersey, a young man who had snorted $100 worth of cocaine every day for six years was about to commit suicide. As he stood on the sixth floor of a parking garage, the image of his young nephew flashed through his mind. Suddenly the man realized that he wanted to send a message to him and to other kids about what drugs can do. Now, he says, "I want to do something about drugs and help other people," perhaps by becoming a drug counselor.

Addiction is a parasite that tries to remain in equilibrium with the host. When I read about this would-be suicide, I could almost visualize a devil standing on one of his shoulders and an angel on the other. Both were whispering in his ear trying to win his soul, and both forces were pretty evenly matched. But I have a gut feeling this guy will make it—his motivation to get better comes from his desire to be of service to others. As he put it, "I think I'm going to be all right. There are things I can do for people." This time, at least, the angel won the tug-of-war.

People who did okay before they got into trouble with drugs—good academic record, steady employment—usually do fine again after they've kicked their habits. Obviously, those who complete an inpatient program and graduate to outpatient follow-up have a better chance than those who quit. If the caregivers do their job and choose the right medical treatment, the patient's choices go up.

To measure success we collect feedback from the patients and their families, friends, and employers. Oh yes—we analyze the patient's urine. Always. Remember: Trust—but verify.

Issues Affecting Therapy

I want to close this chapter with a brief look at some of the problems we face in providing residential care. We'll be wrestling with some of these issues through the end of this decade and beyond.

Most troublesome are the severe shortages in the number of treatment slots available. Since the dawn of crack, many treatment programs, especially those in urban areas, are reportedly full to bursting. Often addicts finally realize they need help and make their way to a treatment program, only to find there's a waiting list—one week, a month, even eight months to a year. But drug users need immediate gratification—after all, that's one reason they use drugs in the first place. A month's wait can seem like a lifetime. And in some cases, it is. In New York recently a woman tried to enter a treatment program but was told she had to wait; a month later she had been murdered. Another young man died of an overdose waiting for a treatment opening.

In this country there are perhaps four million addicts (defined, somewhat arbitrarily, as people who use drugs at least 200 times a year) but only about 600,000 treatment slots. Even if a fourth of our addicts wanted help, we'd still be 400,000 slots short. (To provide treatment to so many addicts, former "Drug Czar" William Bennett's proposal of boot camps for addicts may someday become a large, government-sponsored treatment program.) It's tragic that so many people must wait, left to face continuing suffering, pain, and even death. That's why I campaign so arduously for prevention—better to keep people from becoming addicts than to make them come for help.

Another problem is that many treatment programs were set up decades ago just to help heroin addicts. Now, though, there are probably six times as many people with cocaine problems as there are heroin junkies, yet there is no special place for them to go. And some who do manage to enter a program may complain that they are being treated by people who don't understand the very different nature of cocaine addiction and the therapy it requires. Studies show that when there's a mismatch between the patient and the treatment, only one out of five addicts get better.

Women face a particularly hard road. Only about 50 treatment programs *in the entire country* provide child and obstetric care, or supply needed services such as counseling for sexual abuse. In Massachusetts, so few programs accept women that some women with drug or alcohol problems are sent to jails. Here's the catch-22, though: Because these women are not official "prisoners," they can't take advantage of inmate drug rehabilitation programs! For some awful reason, crack is highly appealing to women, much more so than heroin ever was. Out of nearly ten million drug users (addicts and otherwise), more than half are women; there are about as many female crack smokers as male. In New York City alone, more than half of the 78 treatment programs exclude all pregnant women; 67 percent won't help pregnant women on Medicaid, and 87 percent won't treat the three-time loser: pregnant, on Medicaid, and addicted to crack. Thus the very women who need help most are turned away.

When a pregnant woman uses drugs, we get two addicts for the price of one. That ain't no bargain. It's been estimated that one million drug babies will have been born between 1988 and 1991, and each one of those kids will need up to $100,000 in extra medical care *just during infancy.* That doesn't begin to account for the extra support they'll need during the rest of their lives—additional counseling, special education, schooling, and so on—to repair the damage to their brains, their bodies, and their ability to function within society.

Sometimes I feel frustrated because our society places roadblocks in the way of people who want to get help. Availability of treatment slots is one such block; cost is another. Insurance companies are more likely to cover the costs of inpatient care, even if outpatient treatment would work just as well. Many policies will cover hospital treatment but cover only 50 percent of the costs of outpatient care. Some patients thus prefer to wait and enter already crowded inpatient programs even though they would do fine, and at much lower cost to everybody, as outpatients. For some puzzling reason, insurers see inpatient and outpatient treatment as competing forces, when in reality they are complementary. Ironically, this managed care is helping everyone to see that the continuum of care is complementary. We need both types of treatment, just as we need hammers and saws to build a house.

Many alcohol programs were designed to last 28 days—and what a coincidence! That happens to match *exactly* the maximum hospital stay that most insurance plans agree to pay for alcohol care. But some patients need less, while others need more than just four weeks to rid themselves of decades of addiction. Steve Tyler, lead singer for the rock group Aerosmith, said he was such a "garbage head" that he had to go through *four* month-long programs before he got free of his addictions to alcohol and heroin.

The good news is that the users, their families, and treatment professionals are advocating a change. They want to determine how long a patient should stay in treatment, not by some artificial time-frame, but by the *progress* the patient makes at different stages of the treatment process. This revolutionary way of thinking recognizes one of the hard realities of addiction: Inpatient care is intended to stabilize the sickest patients and get them through the immediate crisis. The hard work—a lifetime of recovery through total abstinence—lies ahead.

As we'll see in the next chapter, that job can be made infinitely easier if the addict gets good support from family and friends.

CHAPTER SIXTEEN

Codependency and Enabling: Treating the Whole Family

Picture an ice-skating rink. As the music plays and the lights sparkle, people glide along in endless circles, everyone moving in the same direction. Some skate smoothly and confidently; a few execute fancy leaps and turns. Others stagger, wobble, and occasionally fall. When that happens, even the most graceful Olympic skater is in danger of colliding with someone else. Everyone benefits if fallen skaters are helped to their feet and shown how to keep moving.

I've used this image because it symbolizes the slippery nature of addiction and its impact on other people—especially the members of the addict's family. At its best, a family is a group of people who help each other learn how to skate through life. If one member of the family suddenly changes direction, or has trouble staying on his or her feet, there's a danger of a collision that could bring everyone down.

Treatment for substance abuse trains recovering addicts to keep their balance. But that treatment doesn't do a damn bit of good if patients then return to a home where they are in great danger of being knocked down, psychologically speaking. Treatment isn't complete, and is thus doomed to fail, unless it shows all other members of the family how to stop acting in ways that only make the addict's problem worse.

Codependency

Part of the good news that has emerged in the past decade is our growing understanding of the role codependency plays in addiction. We define the dependent as the person who has the substance abuse problem. Sometimes we refer to that person as the "identified" addict or patient. Such a phrase implies, correctly, that there are other, unidentified addicts involved—the codependents. A *codependent* is anyone directly involved with the dependent's life—parents, spouse, children, even close friends. They are called codependents because their behavior and attitudes affect the patient, and the patient in turn affects them. The dependent is sick, while codependents belong to a sick family system. Like ice skaters, families are codependent; one person's actions influence everyone else.

Addiction is thus very much a family affair. In Chapter Four we learned how biology influences addiction. The likelihood of substance abuse is determined, to some extent, by the genes we inherit from our parents. Thus even children who are adopted at birth by the healthiest families in the world may still be at risk if one or both of their biological parents were substance abusers.

Here's the sad part: Though they may be completely unaware of it, codependents come to define their roles in life by their relationship to their loved one's addiction. When the addict tries to get help, the family may feel threatened. The "
ance" they've struggled to achieve, a balance whose focal point is the identified patient's addiction, is about to be lost. Thus, tragically, the codependents often interfere with the process of treatment—consciously, through sabotage and denial, or subconsciously, by resisting their own need to change. The dependent is hooked on a chemical, while the *codependents are hooked on their sick family system.*

Cullen, aged 22, had been a cocaine user for seven years. After discovering crack two years ago, he developed a bad case of crack lung: severe chest pains, difficulty breathing, and fever. He missed work so often that he was fired and had to move back to his mother Maura's home. Ironically, although Maura worked as a nurse here at Fair Oaks, she was oblivious to the cause of her son's illness. She was blinded by her delight at having her son return to the nest. As a nurse and a mother, she never felt more needed than now, as she tended to her "poor baby." Since he had no income of his own she gave him her bank card and free access to her accounts. To buy his drugs, Cullen made hundreds of dollars of withdrawals; his mother either failed to keep track or she chose to ignore it. One day she even caught him smoking crack in his bedroom. Rather than pack him off to her own hospital for treatment, she redoubled her efforts as his caretaker. "He just needs more tender loving care," she thought. Maura was a codependent. In order to satisfy her needs as nurse and mother, she wanted her son to stay sick.

Kyle, aged 45, owner of a public relations firm, had known his wife Mia was an alcoholic even before they were married, but he loved her so much he believed he could "save" her. When mommy got so drunk she passed out, he told their two kids she was "tired" and carried her upstairs. He then fed and clothed the kids, drove them to school or football practice or to their piano lessons, and still somehow managed to build up his business. All their friends and family knew about Mia's problem and regarded Kyle as a kind of saint—"Look at him, dealing with that lush of a wife and still able to raise good kids and run a business and never complain. How does he do it?" Finally, after 18 years of this, Mia finally crumbled. She made a suicidal gesture, which, she later acknowledged, was nothing more than a pathetic cry for help. She went through rehabilitation and did very well. Her biggest breakthrough, however, came when she realized how Kyle had resisted helping her get treatment. "He's using my alcoholism to feed his own ego," she said bitterly. Yes, I told her; he is your codependent.

Erika, 19 years old, had abused alcohol and marijuana practically every day for many years. Her parents told me they had known about her habits since she was 15. "What have you done so far to try and help her?" I asked. I could hardly contain my surprise when they replied, "Nothing." They said they were terrified that confronting her about her problem would only make it worse. Erika is high strung, they said; she has a violent temper and she might try to hurt herself if we opposed her. "She's hurting herself now," I said quietly, "and she's hurting you." I saw clearly how Erika had turned her parents into emotional hostages, unable to respond, unable to act, and in danger of losing their ability to feel.

I could go on. In fact, *every case of substance abuse I have ever handled reflects some aspect of codependency to one extent or another.*

Denial

Earlier we saw how denial is one of the inevitable symptoms of dependency. The addicts says, "I don't have a drug problem. I can stop any time. Everybody else has the problem."

But denial is a symptom of codependency as well. Parents say, "Drugs are a phase; all kids go through it. Ours will grow out of it. Better not to rock the boat." Spouses say, "She promised she'd stop tomorrow, or next week, or after the first of the year, or when the pressure lets up at work." It may be strange to think of it, but many employers use denial as well: "I hire only good people; I'm too smart to hire a drug addict. I don't need a drug-testing program in my business." Even doctors deny evidence of drug abuse: "My patient says he only uses drugs because he is under stress. I'll prescribe an antidepressant or an antianxiety drug. That should help. And it will be easier on me than trying to cure him of addiction."

One of the hardest challenges of treatment is convincing codependents that they too must overcome their denial and get help. Often parents will haul their kid into my office and demand that I cure him (or her) of his (or her) addiction. They cry, they moan, they beg: "Please make our precious Jimmy (or Jodi) well." I do my best to reassure these parents that I think my program will help. "Oh thank you, thank you," they say, wiping their eyes. Then I drop the bomb: Part of my prescription requires them to participate in family therapy sessions. Suddenly these parents—so grateful just minutes before—stiffen up and say, in effect, "No thanks. This is Jimmy's (or Jodi's) problem, not ours. We'll just take our business elsewhere."

Strange as it may seem, denial in and of itself is not an intrinsically bad thing. In a sense, it is actually part of our psychic defense against shock, and is thus vital to our survival. Let me explain. Some people who are hurt in, say, a car accident report that their entire body goes numb. The pain is so great, in other words, that the nerves shut down to prevent system overload. Similarly, the mind blanks out the memory of the event. These strategies prevent the physical and mental impact of the trauma from destroying the victim.

Denial works the same way: It temporarily insulates us from shock, thus cushioning the worst of the blow. But eventually denial must be set aside so that the *real* process of healing can begin. Only after victims of trauma begin to feel again can we know if they're getting better. Treatment for addiction must acknowledge the existence of denial, accept that it serves a valuable *but temporary* purpose, and then work to break through it.

The Patterns of Codependency

Having worked with many families of substance abusers, I have seen how certain patterns, or themes, constantly recur. Here are a few of those patterns.

Emotional Anesthesia: This is the same old wine—denial—in a brand new bottle. The dependent's problems get so bad that others in the family simply tune out and quit feeling anything. As I indicated, denial is healthy—to some degree, and for a short time. When emotional numbness becomes the only mechanism for dealing with a problem, it becomes a problem in itself.

Silence Is Golden: Another way of saying this is, "If we don't talk about the problem, maybe it'll go away." Nope, Uh-uh. Sorry. In many ways, addiction is a cry for help. If that cry goes unheeded, it will just get louder.

Business as Usual: By this I mean the codependent family's pattern of sticking to their old bad habits and refusing to budge —even when it's in their own best interests to do so. Again, this pattern is woven from the threads of denial. The thinking goes something like this: "If we admit we have to change our ways, then we are admitting that we made mistakes in the past. But that's hard to accept; it undermines our whole philosophy of living, and casts doubt on everything we've ever done or though or valued as a family. It's easier to stick to our guns and forge on."

Balancing Act: It's a natural human tendency to keep the patterns of our daily lives in balance. We don't like too many shocks or stresses to disrupt the routines we have become comfortable with. Codependents tend to assume the role of "balancers" within the family. A wife who sees her husband's cocaine addiction increasing will in turn try to increase the extent of her control—more monitoring, more criticizing, and more attempts to shield the kids or the outside world from becoming aware of the problem. The more the dependent's substance abuse threatens to wreck the marriage and the family, the harder the codependent struggles to preserve them.

In time, though, such efforts to maintain balance are doomed to fail. Codependents will wind up investing all their energies in trying to keep the dependent happy, and have no energy left over for themselves. Ironically, in their attempt to keep things balanced, codependents eventually surrender all power over their own feelings and behavior to the dependent. On the other hand, some codependents are so enraged that they dominate and humiliate the addicted member of the family. They refuse to give the dependent any responsibility and thus they perpetuate his dependency—not just on a chemical, but on other people as well.

The patterns I've described become so ingrained in a family's internal "programming" that the members begin to act like robots carrying out orders they no longer have the power to resist. Therapy for codependency changes this programming. When treatment works—and in many cases it works beautifully—the effect is the same as when hypnotists snap their fingers and command their subjects to wake up.

Enabling

In many cases codependents cross a dangerous line. They themselves become dependent on preserving the situation involving their substance-abusing relative, unhealthy as that situation may be. When they cross that line, two things happen: The codependents stop actively trying to fight the dependent's habit, and they begin to do things (subconsciously or not) that only make the problem worse. In short, they have become enablers.

Let me explain the concept of enabling by telling you about a case one of my colleagues, Dr. Charles Norris, recently handled at Fair Oaks in Florida. The identified addict was a 21-year-old man named Coby. Having lived with his mother for many years, he had recently decided to move in with his father. Even though Coby was a high school dropout, his father—thrilled at getting his son back—made him an executive in his company. He gave the kid a company car, set him up in a company condominium, and gave him tons of responsibility. Coby was ill-equipped to handle the combination of high pay, fast living, and enormous job pressure. He got hooked on cocaine, began missing work, and screwed up a bunch of big projects.

The father brought Coby in for treatment. When the subject of enabling came up, the father said, "What do you mean? I didn't cause this kid's problem." Dr. Norris asked, "Who pays for his car?" "I do—well, the company does," said dad. "Who pays for his house?" "The company." "If any other of your employees had screwed up this badly, would that person still be working for you?" The father's face changed. "No," he said quietly, "that employee would have been canned long ago." That moment was a breakthrough. From then on, much of Coby's treatment focused on helping the father learn how to stop enabling his son to continue abusing drugs.

Enabling can take many forms—making excuses for the addict, giving him money, or tolerating abuse in the home. I know of some codependents who actually buy the drugs or alcohol and give them to their substance-abusing relative. I am amazed at their rationalizations: "If I take charge of getting the booze, I buy less than he would anyway. This way I can at least control the amount we have in the house." "I buy the crack for her because I don't want her messing with those scumbag dealers—that's dangerous." Other enablers lie, cover up, bail their relatives out of jail, do their kids' homework for them, help them with office work, and drive them places. "It keeps the peace," said one. "It's safer if I do it." "I love her and if I can help her by doing this, I will."

This is a book about good news, but I always give enablers the bad news, and I give it to 'em straight: You are *not* helping anyone this way. Quite the opposite—you are only fueling the fire. Worse, you are at risk yourself. The strain of living with, and covering up for, a drug-using family member can lead to serious mental health problems for others in the household. A survey we did at Fair Oaks revealed that 32 percent of parents and 67 percent of spouses developed depression before they managed to get their dependent relative into treatment.

Part of family treatment. then, is devoted to getting an important message across to the enablers: No more bailouts. No more cover-ups. No more lies. No more "anything goes." We work to empower the enablers to say to the addict, "You may want to go to hell, but I won't let you drag me there with you."

Children of Addicts

To me, among the biggest tragedies of substance abuse is its impact on children. (By children I mean offspring of any age.) Children may carry the burden of their parents' substance abuse from the day they are born to the day they die. Some may become addicts themselves; even those who don't develop an addiction may suffer emotional or physical disorders due to anger or guilt.

There is no clearly etched, well-framed portrait that we can label "Typical Child of a Substance Abuser." Each individual is different. However, we can trace patterns that emerge regularly.

For one thing, the children of addicts suffer from overwhelming shame. When very young, they sense—wrongly, of course—that they are somehow to blame for their parent's condition. They think, "It's all my fault that Daddy drinks so much. If I were a better person, or if I loved him more, or if I tried harder, maybe he wouldn't be sick." Children sense that they have to hide their shame, or they'll just make things worse. One patient told us at Fair Oaks, "In our family there were two rules. The first was, never wash your dirty linen in public. The second was, don't wash it at home either." In other words, don't talk about the Family Problems, either inside the house or out of it. This is the child's-eye view of the "silence is golden" pattern I described earlier.

The child tries to hide such feelings, but they usually emerge in a disguised or distorted form. One form is overwhelming sadness, which may develop into full-blown depression. Another is anger, which may erupt as some form of conduct disorder or antisocial behavior. In their effort to control their feelings, many children of addicts adopt a rigid and inflexible attitude toward the world. This attitude makes it harder for them to ask for help or respond to treatment for their codependency.

As we discussed earlier, parents are a child's first and best teachers. But if the only role model parents provide is that of a substance abuser, the child will see the world from a distorted perspective. Adults have the resources to change their world—either by making it better or by fleeing it altogether. Young children, though, are trapped. The only values and social skills they have are the ones they learn from their parents. And what a sorry bunch of skills they are: dishonesty, distrust, manipulation, seething anger, suppressed resentment, and stony silence.

Children of addicts develop certain predictable personality traits to help them make order out of the chaos that swirls around them. Some children become "heroes" or "superchildren." These are the ones who work hard to get good grades, as if doing so will show the world that all is well at home, that there are no problems. Or they take on the burden of running the house while mommy lies in a sodden stupor on the sofa. These superkids cook, clean, pay bills, tend to their siblings, and lie to employers who call to find out why Joe isn't at his desk. Some even go to work at very young ages to bring more money into the house. These kids are often forced to cross generational boundaries—they act like parents as their parents act like children. They become their parents' confidants and counselors. Those jobs are hard enough for trained professionals; a 13-year-old schoolgirl shouldn't be asked to handle such an enormous burden.

Other kids refuse to cooperate with such a sick system and instead become "scapegoats." These are the children likely to shun the family and run away or act out against the world. Often a "scapegoat" is the sibling of a "hero," and is always being compared unfavorably: "Why can't you get good grades like your sister?" "At least your brother cleans up his room once in a while." Their method of solving their problem with their parents' substance abuse is to divert attention from it. This strategy is no more helpful than setting a fire to distract people from the robbery going on down the street.

The "lost child" is the one who copes with the stress by completely shutting down—the emotional anesthesia I mentioned before. Such a child will refuse to enter into relationships with other people out of mistrust or fear of getting hurt.

They suppress their own ambitions, take meaningless jobs that demand nothing of them, and generally try to make themselves invisible as they pass through life, detached and empty.

The "family mascot" is—well, let me explain by telling you about Don, the son of an alcoholic father. When he was growing up, his family bickered constantly. Money was always tight because Dad couldn't keep a job. Don's mother was a native of France; during World War II she was swept off her feet by the handsome American GI who married her and whisked her back to the United States. Mama harbored fantasies of returning to France; these fantasies grew particularly strong the more her husband got lost in his alcoholic haze. Meanwhile Don did everything he could to keep the family happy. During tense family dinners he would break into endless comedy routines—putting napkins on his head and talking in high squeaky voices; doing imitations of the other family members until they roared with laughter. Even today he finishes virtually every thought with some kind of punch line. Once, in a moment of weakness, with Dad passed out upstairs and his mother weeping in his arms, ten-year-old Don—"my little Donnie"—promised that one day he would take Mama back to France forever. For years afterward, every move Don tried to make to establish his independence—taking a job, moving away, getting married—was nearly thwarted by his mother, who was still waiting for her "funny little boy"—her mascot—to escort her back to her homeland.

Related to the mascot is the "diplomat"—the one who tries to smooth things over, to negotiate among warring family members, who tries to pour oil on the troubled waters.

The children of addicts must wrestle with a whole army of demons: low self-esteem, poor self-awareness, hopelessness, sadness, and shame. While normal children grow up in an atmosphere of loving reassurance and calm stability, the family life of the codependent child is chaotic and unpredictable. Not realizing that they can't be responsible for their parent's problems, they are burdened with enormous guilt for failing to solve them. They feel powerless, insecure, and scared. To compensate they seek to exert control, if not over themselves then over others. They avoid having feelings or expressing them. They may become overresponsible to compensate for their parent's lack of responsibility. They ignore—or perhaps simply cannot recognize—their own emotional needs and feelings.

The children of alcoholics and drug addicts are the true victims of substance abuse.

Recovery

In the past few years I have seen a revolution in the field of treatment for substance abuse. It started with our growing awareness of how drug and alcohol addiction affected not just those who ingested the chemicals but those who had to suffer their emotional and mental side effects as well—the codependents. Therapy is now more effective than ever because it recognizes its obligation to treat the whole person: not just individuals, but their entire social context as well.

A virtual industry has sprung up from this awareness. Today there are many programs, clinical as well as self-help, that address the needs of codependents of any age. For example, the success of Alcoholics Anonymous has led to the creation of Alateen for teenagers, Al-Anon for families of alcoholics, and other groups that focus on adult children of alcoholics (ACOAs). Many of the principles espoused by these alcohol-related programs apply to the treatment of codependents of other types of drug abusers as well.

Many rehabilitation centers offer separate therapy programs for the partners or families of dependents while their loved ones are being cared for, either as outpatients or inpatients. At the Outpatient Recovery Center of Fair Oaks Hospital, for example, we provide treatment that may even begin before the dependent starts his or her own process of rehabilitation.

At Fair Oaks, and at many other clinical centers as well, therapy involves an intensive one-week family intervention. During this phase much time is spent breaking through the wall of denial. The process, frankly, is not easy for anybody—neither the identified addict, the family, nor (I admit) for the therapist. But it must be done. Quite understandably, people find it very hard to admit that they may be contributing to another person's illness: "Drive someone to drink—*moi?*" But unless they recognize that a problem exists and come to terms with their role in perpetuating that problem, neither the identified addict nor the codependents will ever get better.

Once that breakthrough occurs, codependents need to be shown that it's worth the trouble to try to recover, and that doing so is certainly better than not recovering. They will see that treatment can help them overcome the burdens of their past and replace confusion, guilt, and fear with hope and a higher sense of self-esteem.

In our view, families are seen as being addicted to the substance abuser, just as the abuser is addicted to a chemical. We work with families to show them how to discover emotional and mental resources deep within themselves, resources they have suppressed or have long since forgotten they ever had. We encourage them to find a peer group to share their burden with, and teach them to stop reacting to the substance abuser or trying to control his behavior. We call this "healthy selfishness," and it's the only way to interrupt their coaddiction and put an end to their enabling. During sessions at Fair Oaks we make it clear to the codependents that unless they clean up the family act, their relative in treatment down the hall doesn't have a prayer of making a permanent recovery.

Part of our treatment strategy involves individual sessions with the various codependents. We also provide group therapy that allows members to share their experiences and to focus on their feelings about things "here and now." Concentrating on the present allows us to break the common codependent obsession with the past and create hope for a positive future.

We also urge our codependent patients to take advantage of Al-Anon groups, since experience shows these to be tremendously valuable, as adjuncts to professional counseling and as long-term aftercare. By participating, people in these groups become aware that they too are at special risk of developing chemical dependency. Often members learn that the patterns of their past may cause them to feel attracted to people with substance abuse problems. Many children of alcoholics, for example, tend to marry other alcoholics, and have alcoholic children, thus perpetuating the cycle. With support from Al-Anon, they avoid repeating past mistakes, or learn how to correct the mistake if it has already been made. There are even Al-Anon groups that focus particularly on this aspect of the disease.

As I've mentioned, many codependents develop severe emotional or mental illnesses as a result of their decades-long struggle. These people may need private psychotherapy or other support that focuses on their problems intensely and exclusively. Many codependent couples benefit from speaking with a professional marriage counselor as well.

Different treatment centers take different approaches. One program, for example—the Onsite inpatient program in Rapid City, South Dakota—uses family therapy aimed at helping people replace their poor self-images with healthier ones through such techniques as role-playing. The Hazeldon Family Centers, at different locations across the country, proceed on the basis that codependency is an essentially normal reaction to abnormal stress. They emphasize the value of education and help patients through discussions, readings, and lectures.

One day soon we will have developed good standards by which to measure the success of all such programs. Meanwhile, we know that any treatment approach that is based on solid facts about drug abuse and that recognizes the role of the family in perpetuating the addiction can be of great value. The most successful programs are those that recognize the goal of treatment is not to cure codependency, but to begin the lifelong process of recovery.

The good news is, those programs are available and are helping thousands of codependents break their old habits and discover that—even after decades of suffering—happiness can be theirs.

APPENDIX

National Resources

I. Private Organizations and Groups

American Council for Drug Education (ACDE)
204 Monroe Street
Rockville, MD 20850
1 (301) 294-0600
1 (800) 488-DRUG

ACDE is an excellent source of information on drugs and substance abuse. Specific information is available for the general public, physicians, education professionals, or employee-assistance personnel.

Beginning Alcohol and Addictions Basic Education Studies (BABES)
17330 Northland Park Court
Southfield, MI 48075
1 (313) 443-0888
1 (800) 54-BABES

BABES is a primary prevention program intent on giving young children a lifetime of prevention from substance abuse. The program uses materials such as cassettes and puppets to help young children respond to their anti-drug message.

1 (800) COCAINE

800 COCAINE is a 24-hour-a-day, 7-days-a-week, telephone hotline owned and operated by National Medical Enterprises. 800 COCAINE provides information on drug abuse and treatment referrals.

1 (800) HELPLINK

The computer-assisted, toll free, and confidential Fair Oaks Hospital information and referral service.

Just Say No International

1777 North California Blvd
Suite 210
Walnut Creek, CA 94596
1 (415) 939-6666
1 (800) 258-2766

"Just Say No" Clubs are groups of children, seven to 14 years old, who are committed to leading drug-free lives and to making their schools and communities drug-free. Contact Just Say No International for more information on establishing a club in your area.

National Families In Action

2296 Henderson Mill Road, Suite 204
Atlanta, GA 30345
1 (404) 934-6364

The National Families In Action specializes in helping to prevent drug abuse in families and in helping families to form community organizations against drug abuse.

The National Federation of Parents for a Drug-Free Youth (NFP)

P.O. Box 3878
St. Louis, Missouri 63122
1 (314) 968-1322

The National Federation of Parents for a Drug-Free Youth provides support for youth and parent groups across the nation.

Partnership for a Drug-Free America

666 Third Avenue
New York, NY 10017
1 (212) 922-1560

The Partnership provides anti-drug information for business and consumers. Videotapes for consumers and professionals that show powerful anti-drug messages may be ordered by calling (212) 973-3517.

PIA Press
19 Prospect Street
Summit, NJ 07901
1 (908) 277-9191
1 (800) 874-2919

Owned by National Medical Enterprises, PIA Press is an excellent source of substance abuse prevention and treatment information for both the consumer and professional. PIA Press also offers information on a wide range of mental health subjects.

PRIDE (Parent's Resource Institute for Drug Education)
The Hurt Building
Suite 210
50 Hurt Plaza
Atlanta, GA 30303
1 (404) 577-4500
1 (900) 988-7743 (PRIDE's drug information telephone hotline. $1 per minute)

PRIDE, the oldest and largest organization devoted to drug abuse prevention through education, provides drug abuse prevention programs to educators, parents, youth and businesses in the United States and other nations.

Toughlove
P.O. Box 1069
Doylestown, PA 18901
1 (215) 348-7090

A nationaal self-help group for parents, children and communities that emphasizes cooperation, action, initiative, and avoidance of blame.

II. Government Organizations

Alcohol and Drug Abuse Education Program
United States Department of Education
400 Maryland Avenue, SW
Washington, DC 20202-4101
1 (202) 708-5366

This program offers a "school team" approach designed to help schools prevent drug and alcohol abuse. Regional centers are available to provide training and technical assistance to local school districts that apply to this program. In addition, a free copy of the publication, *Growing Up Drug Free* (available in English or Spanish), may be obtained by calling 1 (800) 624-0100.

National Clearinghouse for Drug and Alcohol Information
Information Services
P.O. Box 2345
Rockville, MD 20852
1 (800) SAY-NO-TO (DRUGS)

Distributes pamphlets, fact sheets, and statistics on drug use in America.

National Institute on Alcoholism and Alcohol Abuse (NIAAA)
P.O. Box 2345
Rockville, MD 20852
1 (301) 468-2600

A publication list is available upon request.

National Institute on Drug Abuse
5600 Fishers Lane
Rockville, MD 20857
1 (301) 443-6245
Drug Abuse Information and Treatment Referral Lines:
1 (800) 662-HELP (4357) (English)
1 (800) 66-AYUDA (Spanish)
Drug-Free Workplace Helpline:
1 (800) 843-4971

National Institute on Drug Abuse (NIDA) hotline specialists provide confidential information about treatment programs, support services, and AIDS, and answer questions about drug abuse and addiction.

The Drug-Free Workplace Helpline provides technical assistance to businesses, industries, and unions who wish to develop and implement comprehensive programs for drug free workplaces.

Office of Substance Abuse Prevention
Alcohol, Drug Abuse, and Mental Health Administration
5600 Fishers Lane
Rockwall II
Rockville, MD 20857
1 (301) 443-0365

III. Self-Help Groups

Alanon Family Group (including Alateen)
P.O. Box 862
Midtown Station
New York, NY 10018-6106

This self-help group helps family members and friends cope with the problems of living with an alcoholic or addict.

Adult Children of Alcoholics
P.O. Box 35623
Los Angeles, CA 90035

A self-help group for adults whose childhood was mared by alcoholic or addicted parents.

Alcoholics Anonymous
General Service Office
468 Park Avenue South
New York, NY 10016

Alcoholics Anonymous is a fellowship of men and women who help each other recover from alcohol addiction. The 12 Step recovery program originated by Alcoholics Anonymous is used as a guide by many other self-help groups to help their members recover from drug abuse, eating disorders, and emotional disorders.

Cocaine Anonymous
World Services, Inc.
3740 Overland Avenue/Suite G
Los Angeles, CA 90034
1 (213) 554-2554
1 (800) 347-8998

Cocaine Anonymous is based on the 12 Step recovery program of Alcoholics Anonymous.

International Doctors in Alcoholics Anonymous
1950 Volney Road
Youngstown, OH 44511

International Lawyers in Alcoholics Anonymous
Suite 200
111 Pearl Street
Hartford, CT 06103

Marijuana Smokers Anonymous
135 South Cypress Avenue
Orange, CA 92666

A recovery group using the principles of AA and designed specifically for marijuana abusers.

Narcotics Anonymous
NA World Services
P.O. Box 9999
Van Nuys, CA 91409
1 (818) 780-3951

Originating in 1953, NA is one of the largest community-based organizations of recovering drug addicts.

National Association for Children of Alcoholics
31706 Coast Highway, Suite 201
South Laguna, CA 92677

BIBLIOGRAPHY

Adams, Edgar H., Gfroerer, Joseph C. "Elevated Risk of Cocaine Use in Adults." *Psychiatric Annals,* Sept. 1988, pp. 527–623.

Addenbrooke, WM, and Rathod, NH., "Relationship Between Waiting Time and Retention in Treatment Amongst Substance Abusers." *Drug and Dependence,* 26 (1990), p. 255–264.

Adler, Jerry. "Hour by Hour Crack." *Newsweek,* Nov. 28, 1988, pp. 64–79.

Alcohol and Drug Abuse Education Program. *An Overview of the School Team Approach,* U.S. Department of Education, 1984.

The American Psychiatric Association Commission on Psychiatric Therapies. *The Somatic Therapies.* American Psychiatric Association, Washington DC, (n.d.), p. 31–50.

Annitto, William J. and Gold, Mark S., "Treating the 'High and Mighty' and the 'Mighty High'." Chapter 16, *Dual Diagnosis,* Slaby, AE, ed. New York: Marcel Dekker, 1991.

Appel, Carmen B. "A Winning Team." *Employee Assistance,* Oct. 1989, pp. 23–25.

Associated Press. "College Didn't Smoke Out the Drug Users." *The Bergen Record,* Nov. 5, 1989, p. 1–7.

Associated Press, "New Government Study Questions Proposed Link to Alcoholism," *The Star-Ledger,* Dec. 26, 1990, P.B.

Associated Press, "U.S. Almost Triples Estimate of Hard-Core Cocaine Users," *The New York Times,* February 7, 1991, p. D24.

Atkinson, Roland M., ed. *Alcohol and Drug Abuse in Old Age.* Washington, D.C.: American Psychiatric Press, 1984, pp. 1–21.

Baker, James N. "Crack Invades the Hamptons." *Newsweek,* June 20, 1988.

Barden, J. C. "Crack Smoking Seen as a Peril to the Lungs." *The New York Times,* Dec. 24, 1989, p. 19.

Bennett, William J. "Fighting Back: Profiles of Citizen and Community Efforts That Are Helping America Win the War on Drugs." Dec. 26, 1989.

Berger, Joseph. "Judgment Replaces Fear in Drug Lessons." *The New York Times,* Oct. 30, 1989, pp. A1, A12.

Berke, Richard L. "Can the Rich and Famous Talk America Out of Drugs?" *The New York Times,* (Nov. 12, 1989), p. E5.

Berke, Richard L. "President's 'Victory Over Drugs' Is Decades Away, Officials Say." *The New York Times,* Sept. 24, 1989, pp. A1, A20.

Bishop, Katherine. "Neighbors in West Use Small Claims Court to Combat Drugs." *The New York Times,* Oct. 17, 1989, p. A15.

Black, Gordon S. *The Attitudinal Basis of Drug Use—1987-1990.* Reports from The Media-Advertising Partnership for a Drug-Free America, Inc., Rochester, NY: The Gordon S. Black Corporation.

Black, Gordon S. *Changing Attitudes Toward Drug Use—1988-1990.* Reports from The Media-Advertising Partnership for a Drug-Free America, Inc., Rochester, NY: The Gordon S. Black Corporation.

Black, Gordon S. *Reports from The Media-Advertising Partnership for a Drug-Free America, Inc.* The Gordon S. Black Corporation.

Black, Gordon S. *Statistical Report.* Reports from The Media-Advertising Partnership for a Drug-Free America, Inc. Rochester, NY: The Gordon S. Black Corporation, July 11, 1988-September 1990.

Black, Gordon S. and Black, Aaron E. "How to Win the Drug War at Home." (Rochester, New York) *Times-Union,* Sept. 22, 1989.

Brain, Paul F., Coward, Gary A. "A Review of the History, Actions, and Legitimate Uses of Cocaine." *Journal of Substance Abuse,* Vol. I (1989), pp. 431–451.

Browne, Malcolm W. "Problems Loom in Effort to Control Use of Chemicals for Illicit Drugs." *The New York Times,* Oct. 24, 1989, pp. C1, C16.

Buckley, William F. "Drug Czar's Rap at Foes not Sweet." (New York) *Daily News,* Dec. 17, 1989, p. 53.

Bylinsky, Gene. "The Inside Story of the Brain." *Fortune,* Dec. 3, 1990, p. 87.

Cadoret, Remi J., Cain, Colleen A., Crowe, Raymond R. "Evidence for Gene-environment Interaction in the Development of Adolescent Antisocial Behavior." *Behavior Genetics,* Vol. 13; No. 3 (1983), pp. 301–310.

Califano, Joseph A., Jr. "Drug War: Fool's Errand No. 3." *The New York Times,* Dec. 8, 1989, p. 39.

Carson, Doyle I. "Still Too Few Psychiatric Services for Teens." *American Medical News,* Sept. 22/29, 1989, pp. 32–33.

Casazza, J. P., Freitas, J., Stambuk D., et al. "The Measurement of D, L-2,3-Butanediol in Controls and Patients with Alcohol Cirrhosis." *Advances in Alcohol and Substance Abuse,* Vol. 7, Nov. 3/4 (1988), pp. 33–35.

Cavazos, Lauro F. "Drug Use Threatens Educational Goals." *Schools Without Drugs: The Challenge,* May/June 1989, pp. 4–6.

Challenge Network. *Schools Without Drugs: The Challenge,* Mar./Apr. 1989, p. 12.

Church, George J. "Fighting Back." *Time,* Sept. 11, 1989, pp. 12–13.

Ciraulo, Domenic A., Barnhill, Jamie G., Ciraulo, Ann Marie, et al. "Parental Alcoholism as a Risk Factor in Benzodiazepine Abuse: A Pilot Study." *American Journal of Psychiatry,* Oct. 10, 1989, pp. 1333–1335.

"Clean for a Day," *The Bergen Record,* Oct. 13, 1989, p. 2.

Cloninger, C. Robert, Igvardsson, Soren, Gilligan, Sheila B., et al. "Genetic Heterogeneity and the Classification of Alcoholism." *Advances in Alcohol and Substance Abuse,* Vol. 7, No. 3/4 (1988).

"Cocaine Lies to You, Makes You Irrational [Interview with Mark Gold]." *USA Today,* Dec. 6, 1989, p. 13A.

Cocores, J. *800-COCAINE Guide to Alcohol and Drug Recovery.* New York: Villard Books, 1990.

Cohen, Sidney. "Cocaine: Acute Medical and Psychiatric Complications." *Psychiatric Annals,* Oct. 1984, pp. 747–749.

Coleman, Chrisena A. "Cosby's Personal Drug Story." *The Bergen Record,* Nov. 2, 1989, p. E14.

Collins, Gregory B., "Drug and Alcohol Use and Addiction Among Physicians," Chapter 52 in *Comprehensive Handbook of Drug*

Addiction, Miller, NS, ed. New York: Marcel Dekker, 1991.

Commission to Deter Criminal Activity. *Don't Get Caught with Drugs Here.* Drug-Free School Zone Brochure, Commission to Deter Criminal Activity, Trenton, NJ.

Comprehensive Approach Yields Success in Bedford-Stuyvesant." *Schools Without Drugs: The Challenge.* Sept./Oct. 1989, p. 13.

Conrad, Scott, Hughes, Patrick, Baldwin, DeWitt C., et al. "Cocaine Use by Senior Medical Students." *American Journal of Psychiatry,* March 1989, pp. 382–383.

Corcoran, David. "Legalizing Drugs: Failures Spur Debate." *The New York Times,* Nov. 27, 1989, p. A15.

"Crack Brained [Editorial]." *The New York Times,* Nov. 6, 1989, p. A22.

"Crack Mothers, Crack Babies and Hope [Editorial]." *The New York Times,* Dec. 31, 1989, p. 38.

Criminal Justice Information System, Research and Systems Division. *Graphs and Charts of Drug Case Statistical Data.* Administrative Office of the Courts.

Culhane, Charles, "Marijuana's Brain Receptor Found," *U.S. Journal,* December 1990, p. 11.

Cushman, John H., Jr. "Private Transportation Workers to Join Ranks of Those Tested for Drug Use." *The New York Times,* Dec. 18, 1989, p. D9.

Dackis, Charles A., Gold, Mark S. "Alcoholism," in *Advances in Psychopharmacology: Predicting and Improving Treatment Response,* Gold, Mark S., Lydiard, R. Bruce, Carman, John S., eds. Boca Raton, Florida: CRC Press, 1986, pp. 227–288.

Dackis, Charles A., Gold, Mark S. "Biological Aspects of Cocaine Addiction," in *Cocaine in the Brain,* Volkow, N. D., ed. New Brunswick, NJ: Rutgers University Press, 1988.

Dackis, Charles A., Gold, Mark S. "Bromocriptine as Treatment of Cocaine Abuse." *The Lancet,* May 18, 1985, pp. 1151–1152.

Dackis, Charles A., Gold, Mark S. "New Concepts in Cocaine Addiction: The Dopamine Depletion Hypothesis." *Neuroscience and Biobehavioral Reviews,* Vol. 9 (1985), pp. 469–477.

Dackis, Charles A., Gold, Mark S. "Pharmacological Approaches to Cocaine Addiction." *Journal of Substance Abuse Treatment,* Vol. 2 (1985), pp. 139–145.

Dackis, Charles A., Gold, Mark S. "Psychopharmacology of Cocaine." *Psychiatric Annals,* Sep. 1988, pp. 528–530.

Dackis, Charles A., Gold, Mark S. "Treatment Strategies for Cocaine Detoxification," unpublished.

Dackis, Charles A., Gold, Mark S., Estroff, Todd W. "Inpatient Treatment of Addiction." *Treatment of Psychiatric Disorders: A Task Force Report of the American Psychiatric Association.* Washington, D.C.: American Psychiatric Association, 1989, pp. 1359–1379.

Dackis, Charles A., Gold, Mark S., Pottash, A.L.C. "Central Stimulant Abuse: Neurochemistry and Pharmacotherapy." *Advances in Alcohol and Substance Abuse,* Vol. 6, No. 2 (1987), pp. 7–21.

Dackis, Charles A., Gold, Mark S., Sweeney, Donald R., et al. "Single-Dose Bromocriptine Reverses Cocaine Craving." *Psychiatry Research,* Vol. 20 (1987), pp. 261–264.

DeMilio, Lawrence, Gold, Mark S., Martin, David. "Evaluation of the Substance Abuser," in *Diagnostic and Laboratory Testing in Psychiatry,* Gold, Mark S., Pottash, A.L.C., eds. New York: Plenum Medical Book Company, 1986, pp. 235–247.

The Diagram Group. *The Brain: A User's Manual.* New York: Berkley Books, 1983.

Diesenhouse, Susan. "Drug Treatment Is Scarcer Than Ever for Women." *The New York Times,* Jan. 7, 1990, p. E26.

"Drug-Free Schools Commission Appointed to Advise on Strategy." *Schools Without Drugs: The Challenge,* Sept./Oct. 1989, p. 11

"Drug Study Finds Regional Bias." *USA Today,* Nov. 6, 1989.

"Drugs: Where We Stand." *Playboy,* May 1987.

Drug Testing in the Workplace, May 1988 Survey, 800-COCAINE.

"Drug Wars Made This Year Bloody." *The Bergen Record,* Dec. 28, 1989.

Eckardt, Michael J., Rohrbaugh, John W., Rio, Daniel, et al. "Brain Imaging in Alcohol Patients." *Advances in Alcohol and Substance Abuse,* Vol. 7, No. 3/4 (1988), pp. 59–71.

Editors of *Playboy.* "Addiction and Rehabilitation." *Playboy,* May 1987.

Edwards, Cary. "Sign of the Times—Drug-Free N.J." *Message from the Office of Attorney General.* New Jersey Department of Law and Public Safety, Trenton, NJ.

Egan, Timothy. "Drug War Weapon: Manpower on Bikes." *The New York Times,* Jan. 3, 1990, p. A16.

Ehrenkranz, Joel R., Hembree, Wylie C. "Effects of Marijuana on Male Reproductive Function." *Psychiatric Annals,* April 1986, pp. 243–248.

Estroff, Todd W. "Chronic Medical Complications of Drug Abuse." *Psychiatric Medicine,* Vol. 3, No. 3 (1987), pp. 267–286.

Estroff, Todd W., Gold, Mark S. "Medical and Psychiatric Complications of Cocaine Abuse with Possible Points of Pharmacological Treatment." *Advances in Alcohol and Substance Abuse,* Vol. 5, No. 1/2 (1986), pp. 61–76.

Estroff, Todd W., Gold, Mark S. "Psychiatric Presentation of Marijuana Abuse." *Psychiatric Annals,* April 1986, pp. 221–224.

Extein, Irl L. "An Update on Cocaine." *Currents,* Feb. 1988, pp. 5–13.

Extein, Irl L., Allen, S. S., Gold, Mark S., et al. "Bromocriptine Versus Desipramine in Cocaine Withdrawal." *APA New Research,* NR264: 130; 1988.

Extein Irl L., Dackis, Charles A., Gold, Mark S., Pottash, A.L.C. "Depression in Drug Addicts and Alcoholics," in *Medical Mimics of Psychiatric Disorders,* Extein, Irl, Gold, Mark S., eds., Washington, D.C.: American Psychiatric Press, 1986, pp. 131–162.

Extein, Irl L., Gold, Mark S. "The Treatment of Cocaine Addicts: Bromocriptine or Desipramine." *Psychiatric Annals,* Sept. 1988, pp. 535–537.

"Fallen Idol." *The Bergen Record,* Nov. 8, 1989, p. A2.

Farber, M. A., Terry, Don. "Out-of-Towners Find New York City a Drug Bazaar." *The New York Times,* Dec. 3, 1989, pp. A1, 56.

Feingold, Barry C. "Deterring Damage." *Employee Assistance,* Oct. 1989, pp. 29–30.

Finlayson, Richard E. "Prescription Drug Abuse in Older Persons," in *Alcohol and Drug Abuse in Old Age,* Atkinson, Roland M., ed. Washington, D.C. American Psychiatric Press, 1984, pp. 62–70.

Fischman, M. W., Foltin, R. W., Nestadt, G., et al. "Effects of Desipramine Maintenance on Cocaine Self-administration by Humans," *Journal of Pharmacology and Experimental Therapeutics,* 253: 760–770; 1990.

Fisher, Lawrence M. "Old Standby, the Corner Bar, Falling Victim to New Values." *The New York Times,* Nov. 18, 1989, p. 1.

"Florida Bus Searches for Drugs Are Ruled Intrusive." *The New York Times,* Dec. 3, 1989, p. 56.

"Forcing Drug Dealers to Really Pay for Their Crime [Editorial]." *Boston Herald,* Nov. 15, 1989, p. 38.

Foster, Willard O. "Integrating Work-Based Policies." *EAP Digest,* Sept./Oct. 1989, pp. 33–41.

Freitag, Michael. "Fears of Neighbors Frustrate a Drug-Care Center." *The New York Times,* Nov. 13, 1989, p. B2.

" 'Frequent Drinker' Offer Stirs Up Spirited Debate." *The Wall Street Journal,* Nov. 1, 1989, p. B5.

Freudenheim, Milt. "More Aid for Addicts on the Job." *The New York Times,* Nov. 13, 1989, pp. D1, D4.

"Future Blueprint." *Employee Assistance,* Oct. 1989, pp. 37–38.

Galanter, Marc. "Management of the Alcoholic in Office Practice." *Psychiatric Annals,* May 1989, pp. 266–270.

Gawin, Frank H., Ellinwood, E. H., Jr. "Cocaine and Other Stimulants." *The New England Journal of Medicine,* May 5, 1988, pp. 1173–1182.

Gawin, Frank H., Kleber, H. D., Byck, R., et al. "Desipramine Facilitation of Initial Cocaine Abstinence," *Archives of General Psychiatry,* 147: 655–657; 1990.

Gold, Mark S. "Crack Abuse: Its Implications and Outcomes." *Resident and Staff Physician,* July 1987, pp. 45–53.

Gold, Mark S. "Dangers in Young People Smoking Pot." *Physician and Patient,* Jan. 1983, pp. 50–52.

Gold, Mark S. *Drugs of Abuse: A Comprehensive Series for Clinicians. Volume I. Marijuana.* New York: Plenum Medical Book Company, 1989.

Gold, Mark S. "Legalize Drugs: Just Say Never," *The National Review,* April 1, 1990, pp. 42–59.

Gold, Mark S. "Medical Implications of Cocaine Intoxication," *Alcoholism and Addiction,* Oct. 1989, p. 16.

Gold, Mark S. *1988 Medical and Health Annual.* Chicago: Encyclopedia Britannica, Inc., 1988, pp. 277–284.

Gold, Mark S. *1987 Medical and Health Annual.* Chicago: Encyclopedia Britannica, Inc., 1987, pp. 184–203.

Gold, Mark S. "The Cocaine Epidemic: What Are the Problems, Insights, and Treatments?" *Pharmacy Times,* Mar. 1987, pp. 36–42.

Gold, Mark S. *The Facts About Drugs and Alcohol, Third Revised Edition.* New York: Bantam Books, 1988.

Gold, Mark S., Dackis, Charles A., Washton, Arnold M. "The Sequential Use of Clonidine and Naltrexone in the Treatment of Opiate Addicts." *Advances in Alcohol and Substance Abuse,* Spring 1984, pp. 19–39.

Gold, Mark S., Estroff, Todd W. "The Comprehensive Evaluation of Cocaine and Opiate Abusers," in *Handbook of Psychiatric Diag-*

nostic Procedures, Vol. 2, Hall, R.C.W., Beresford, T. P., eds. Costa Mesa, CA: PMA Publishing Corp., 1985, pp. 213–230.

Gold, Mark S., Estroff, Todd W., Pottash, A.L.C. "Substance Induced Organic Mental Disorders," in *Psychiatry Update: American Psychiatric Association Annual Review, Vol. 4,* Hales, Robert E., and Frances, Allen J., eds.: Washington: American Psychiatric Press, 1985, pp. 227–240.

Gold, Mark S., et al. *Stop Drugs at Work.* New York: Random House Professional Business Publications, 1986.

Gold, Mark S., Fox, Corinne Frantz. "Antianxiety and Opiates." *The Behavioral and Brain Sciences,* Sept. 1982, pp. 486–487.

Gold, Mark S. (moderator), Frances, Richard J., Washton, Arnold M., et al. "Roundtable: People Who Use Illicit Drugs at Work." *Medical Aspects of Human Sexuality,* Oct. 1985.

Gold, Mark S., Pottash, A.L.C. "Endorphins, Locus Coeruleus, Clonidine, and Lofexidine: A Mechanism for Opiate Withdrawal and New Nonopiate Treatments." *Advances in Alcohol and Substance Abuse,* Fall 1981, pp. 33–51.

Gold, Mark S., Pottash, A.L.C., Annitto, William J., et al. "Cocaine Withdrawal: Efficacy of Tyrosine (Abstract)." *Society for Neuroscience 13th Annual Meeting,* Boston: Nov. 6–11, 1983, p. 157.

Gold, Mark S., Pottash, A.L.C., Annitto, William J., et al. "Lofexidine: A Clonidine Analogue Effective in Opiate Withdrawal." *The Lancet,* May 2, 1981, pp. 992–993.

Gold, Mark S., Pottash, A.L.C., Annitto, William J., Vereby, Karl. "Efficacy of Naltrexone in Opiate Addiction." *Syllabus and Scientific Proceedings, Annual Meeting.* New York: American Psychiatric Association Continuing Medical Education, 1983, pp. 267–268.

Gold, Mark S., Pottash, A.L.C., Extein, Irl. "Clonidine: Inpatient Studies from 1978–1981." *Journal of Clinical Psychiatry,* June 1982, pp. 35–38.

Gold, Mark S., Pottash, A.L.C., Extein, Irl. "From Opiate Addiction Naltrexone Via Clonidine." *Syllabus and Scientific Proceedings, Annual Meeting.* American Psychiatric Association Continuing Medical Education, New York: 1982, p. 126.

Gold, Mark S., Pottash, A.L.C., Percel, Joseph, et al. "Naltrexone in the Treatment of Physician Addicts." *Syllabus and Scientific Proceedings, Annual Meeting.* American Psychiatric Association Continuing Medical Education, New York: 1982, p. 275.

Gold, Mark S., Pottash, A.L.C., Sweeney, Donald R., et al. "Lofexidine Blocks Acute Opiate Withdrawal," in *Problems of Drug Dependence, 1981: Proceedings of the 43rd Annual Scientific Meeting, The Committee on Problems of Drug Dependence, Inc.,* Harris, Louis S., ed. NIDA research monograph 41, April 1982, pp. 264–268.

Gold, Mark S., Pottash, A.L.C., Sweeney, Donald R., et al. "Opiate Detoxification with Lofexidine." *Drug and Alcohol Dependence,* Vol. 8 (1981), pp. 307–315.

Gold, Mark S., Redmond, D. E., Jr., Kleber, H. D. "Clonidine May Relieve Opiate Withdrawal Symptoms," *Journal of the American Medical Association,* 240(23): 2557; 1978.

Gold, Mark S., Slaby, A. E., eds. *Dual Diagnosis in Substance Abuse.* New York: Marcel Dekker, Inc., 1991.

Gold, Mark S., Verebey, Karl. "The Psychopharmacology of Cocaine." *Psychiatric Annals,* Oct. 1984, pp. 714–723.

Gold, Mark S., Washton, Arnold M., Dackis, Charles A. "Cocaine Abuse: Neurochemistry, Phenomenology, and Treatment," in *National Institute on Drug Abuse Research Monograph Series 61,* Kozel, Nicholas J., Adams, Edgar H., eds. Rockville, MD: NIDA, 1985, pp. 130–150.

Gold, Mark S., Washton, Arnold M., Dackis, Charles A., Chatlos, J. Calvin. "New Treatments for Opiate and Cocaine Users: But What About Marijuana?" *Psychiatric Annals,* April 1986, pp. 206–214.

Goodwin, Donald W., Schulsinger, Fini, Knop, Joachim, et al. "Alcoholism and Depression in Adopted-Out Daughters of Alcoholics." *Archives of General Psychiatry,* July 1977, pp. 751–755.

Googins, Bradley K. "Opening the Black Box." *Employee Assistance,* Oct. 1989, p. 10.

Gould, Alan D. "New Weapon Against Drugs: A Stamp Tax (Editorial)." *The New York Times,* Jan. 1990, p. 25.

Grady, Sandy. "Bailing Out the Atlantic by Bucket (Editorial)." *The Bergen Record,* Dec. 18, 1989.

Grant, Igor, Adams, Kenneth M., Reed, Robert. "Intermediate-Duration (Subacute) Organic Mental Disorder of Alcoholism," in *Neuropsychiatric Correlates of Alcoholism,* Grant, Igor, ed. Washington, D.C.: American Psychiatric Press, 1986, pp. 38–60.

Greenhouse, Linda. "Chief Justice Makes Plea for More Federal Judgeships to Help in Fight Against Drugs." *The New York Times,* Jan. 1990, p. 10.

Greve, Frank. "Phoenix's Hard Line on Casual Drug Use." *The Bergen Record,* Nov. 24, 1989, p. A26.

Gross, Jane. "Grandmothers Bear a Burden Sired by Drugs." *The New York Times,* Apr. 9, 1989, p. A1.

Harrison, Bruce S., Simpler, Gary L. "Antidrug Rules and Regulations." *EAP Digest,* Sept./Oct. 1989, pp. 19–24.

Hays, Constance L. "Police Chief Quits in Massachusetts." *The New York Times,* Nov. 4, 1989.

Henricks, Lorraine. *Kids Who Do/Kids Who Don't: A Parent's Guide to Teens and Drugs.* Summit, New Jersey: PIA Press, 1989, pp. 14–17.

Herridge, Peter, Gold, Mark S. "Pharmacological Adjuncts in the Treatment of Opioid and Cocaine Addicts." *Journal of Psychoactive Drugs,* July-Sept. 1988, pp. 233–242.

Herridge, Peter, Gold, Mark S. "The New User of Cocaine: Evidence from 800-COCAINE." *Psychiatric Annals,* Sep. 1988, pp. 521–522.

HHS News. Press release, July 31, 1989.

Hong, Robert, Matsuyama, Eugene, and Nur, Khalid. "Cardiomyopathy Associated With the Smoking of Crystal Methamphetamine." *Journal of the American Medical Association,* March 6, 1991, Vol. 265, No. 9, pp. 1152–54.

"Household Survey Shows Declining Drug Use Nationwide." *Schools Without Drugs: The Challenge,* Sept./Oct. 1989, p. 7.

"How Do You Say No?" *Schools Without Drugs: The Challenge,* May/June 1989, p. 11.

"How to Help Win the Drug War." *Your Health,* Nov. 21, 1989, reprinted from *U.S. News and World Report.*

Hyman, Steven E. "An Update on Molecular Genetics in Psychiatry." *Currents,* 1989.

Intoxication Levels Are Rising for Students Using Drugs in U. S. Press release from PRIDE, Sept. 26, 1989.

Irwin, Michael, Schuckit, Marc A. "Neurophysiologic and Psychologic Characteristics of Men at Risk for Alcoholism." in *Neuropsychiatric Correlates of Alcoholism,* Grant, Igor, ed. Washington, D.C.: American Psychiatric Press, 1986, pp. 2–20.

Judge, William J., Evans, David. "Drug-Testing Decisions: Implications for EAPs." *EAP Digest,* Sep./Oct. 1989, pp. 25–32.

Kelley, Jack. "Poll: Drug Crisis Worse Than Realized." *USA Today,* Oct. 24, 1989, p. A1.

Khantzian, E. J., Khantzian, N.J. "Cocaine Addiction: Is There a Psychological Predisposition?" *Psychiatric Annals,* Vol. 14, No. 10 (1984), pp. 753–759.

Kilpatrick, James J. "Drug War Has Yet to Start [Editorial]." *The Bergen Record,* Nov. 24, 1989, p. A51.

Kilpatrick, James J. "Let's Just Say No—to Legalizing Drugs [Editorial]." *The Bergen Record,* Dec. 17, 1989, p. O4.

Kleber, Herbert D., "Federal Drug Plan Targets Many Issues." *U.S. Journal,* March 1991, p. 5.

Kline, David. "The Anatomy of Addiction." *Equinox,* Sep./Oct. 1985, pp. 77–86.

Kolata, Gina. "Drug Researchers Try to Treat a Nearly Unbreakable Habit." *The New York Times,* June 25, 1988, pp. 1, 30.

Kolata, Gina. "Study Tells Why Alcohol Is Greater Risk to Women." *The New York Times,* Jan. 10, 1990, pp. A1, D22.

Kraar, Louis. "The Drug Trade." *Fortune,* June 20, 1988, pp. 27–38.

Kupfer, Andrew. "What To Do About Drugs." *Fortune,* June 20, 1988, pp. 39–41.

Labaton, Stephen. "Federal Judge Urges Legalization of Crack, Heroin and Other Drugs." *The New York Times,* Dec. 13, 1989, pp. A1, B10.

Labaton, Stephen. "The Cost of Drug Abuse: $60 billion a year." *The New York Times,* Dec. 5, 1989, pp. D1, D6.

Lacayo, Richard. "On the Front Lines." *Time,* Sep. 11, 1989, pp. 14–18.

Lamar, Jacob V. "Kids Who Sell Crack." *Time,* May 9, 1988, pp. 20–33.

Lerner, Michael A. "The Fire of 'Ice.'" *Newsweek,* Nov. 27, 1989, pp. 37–40.

Light, Kim. "Drug-Free Schools Conference Highlights State, Local Programs." *Schools Without Drugs: The Challenge,* May/June 1989, pp. 1, 3, 6.

Linnoila, Markku. "Neurotransmitters and Alcoholism: Methodological Issues." *Advances in Alcohol and Substance Abuse,* Vol 7, No. 3/4 (1988), pp. 17–24.

"Liquor Consumption in U.S. Reported at a 3-Decade Low." *The New York Times,* Nov. 25, 1989.

Macdonald, Donald Ian, Cechowiz, Dorynne. "Marijuana: A Pediatric Overview." *Psychiatric Annals,* April 1986, pp. 215–218.

Magnuson, Ed. "Bright Kids, Bad Business." *Time,* Sep. 11, 1989, p. 18.

Magyar, Mark J. "Sign of the Times: 'Drug-Free Block.'" *The Bergen Record* (Nov. 28, 1989), p. A1.

Malcolm, Andrew H. "Crack, Bane of Inner City, Is Now Gripping Suburbs." *The New York Times,* Oct. 1989, pp. A1, A24.

Malcolm, Andrew H. "In Making Drug Strategy, No Accord on Treatment." *The New York Times,* Nov. 19, 1989, pp. A1, 34.

Malcolm, Andrew H. "More Americans Are Killing Each Other." *The New York Times,* Dec. 31, 1989, p. A20.

"Management Survey Identifies Substance Abuse as Nation's Number One Workplace Issue." *AMHA Newsletter,* Nov. 1989, pp. 6–7.

Mariott, Michel. "Addicts Awaiting Treatment Often Face Delays and Panic." *The New York Times,* Jan. 9, 1990, pp. A1, B4.

Marriott, Michel. "A Pioneer in Residential Drug Treatment Reaches Out." *The New York Times,* Nov. 13, 1989, p. B2.

Marriott, Michel. "Struggle and Hope from Ashes of Drugs." *The New York Times,* Oct. 22, 1989, pp. A1, 36.

Martz, Larry. "A Tide of Drug Killing." *Newsweek,* Jan. 16, 1989, pp. 44–45.

Max, B. "This and That: Chocolate Addiction, the Dual Pharmacogenetics of Asparagus Eaters, and the Arithmetic of Freedom." *TiPS,* Oct. 1989, pp. 390–393.

McKinley, James C., Jr. "Brooklyn Teen-Ager Killed for Failing to Give a High-5." *The New York Times,* Jan. 10, 1990, p. B3.

McKinley, James C., Jr. "Gunmen Kill 2 Bystanders in 'Power Play'." *The New York Times,* Dec. 27, 1989, p. B1.

McQueen, Michel, Shribman, David. "Battle Against Drugs Is Chief Issue Facing Nation, Americans Say." *The Wall Street Journal,* Sep. 22, 1989, pp. 1, 14.

Meddis, Sam. "War on Drugs Is Lost; Let's Seek New Ideas." *USA Today,* Oct. 30, 1989, p. 11A.

Meyer, Anne. "Parents and Schools: An Important Partnership in the War on Drugs." *Schools Without Drugs: The Challenge,* Mar./Apr. 1989, pp. 7, 10.

Milam, James R., Ketcham, Katherine. *Under the Influence: A Guide to the Myths and Realities of Alcoholism.* New York: Bantam Books, 1983.

Miller, Norman, Gold, Mark S. "Cocaine and Alcoholism: Distinct or Part of a Spectrum?" *Psychiatric Annals,* Sept. 1988, pp. 538–539.

Miller, Norman S., Gold, Mark S. *Drugs of Abuse: A Comprehensive Series for Clinicians. Volume II.* New York: Plenum Medical Book Company, 1991.

Miller, Norman S., Gold, Mark S. "The Medical Diagnosis and Treatment of Alcohol Dependence." *Resident and Staff Physician.* 36 (10): 73–81, 1990.

Miller, Norman S., Gold, Mark S. "Research Approaches to Inheritance to Alcoholism." *Substance Abuse* (In Press).

Miller, Norman S., Gold, Mark S. "Suggestions for Changes in DSM-III-R Criteria for Substance Use Disorders." *American Journal of Drug and Alcohol Abuse,* Vol. 15, No. 2 (1989) pp. 223–230.

Miller, Norman S., Gold, Mark S., Pottash, A. L. C. "A 12-Step Approach for Marijuana (cannabis) Dependence." *Journal of Substance Abuse Treatment,* 6 (4): 241–250, 1989.

Miller, Norman S., Gold, Mark S., Pottash, A.L.C., "Reports from Research Centers—Fair Oaks Clinical Research Center." *British Journal of Addiction,* (86), 1989, pp. 599–606.

Miller, Norman S., Mirin, Steven M. "Multiple Drug Use in Alcoholics: Practical and Theoretical Implications." *Psychiatric Annals,* May 1989, pp. 248–255.

Mirin, Steven M. "Alcoholism: Some Cause for Optimism." *Psychiatric Annals,* May 1989, p. 235.

Mirin, Steven M., ed. *Substance Abuse and Psychopathology.* Washington, D.C.: Clinical Insights: The Monograph Series of the American Psychiatric Press, Inc., 1984, pp. 20–40.

Mirin, Steven M., Weiss, Roger D. "Genetic Factors in the Development of Alcoholism." *Psychiatric Annals,* May 1989, pp. 239–242.

Mitchell, John. "Chemical Balance." *Employee Assistance,* Oct. 1989, pp. 12–17 ff.

Moore, Mark H. "Actually, Prohibition Was a Success [Editorial]." *The New York Times,* Oct. 16, 1989, p. A21.

Mulé, S. Joseph. "The Pharmacodynamics of Cocaine Abuse." *Psychiatric Annals,* Oct. 1984, pp. 724–727.

Munjack, Dennis J., Moss, Howard B. "Affective Disorder and Alcoholism in Families of Agoraphobics." *Archives of General Psychiatry,* Aug. 1981, pp. 869–871.

Nace, Edgar P. "Personality Disorder in the Alcohol Patient." *Psychiatric Annals,* May 1989, pp. 256–260.

National Institute of Justice. *DUF: Drug Use Forecasting, January to March 1989.* U.S. Department of Justice, Office of Justice Programs, Sept. 1989.

National Institute on Alcohol Abuse and Alcoholism. *Alcohol and*

Health, The Seventh Special Report to the U.S. Congress. U.S. Department of Health and Human Services, Publication No. (ADM) 90-1656, Rockville, MD, January 1990.

National Institute on Drug Abuse. *Statistical Series: Semiannual report: Trend data Through July–December 1988.* Data from the Drug Abuse Warning Network, Series G., Number 23, Rockville, MD, p. 8 ff.

National Institute on Drug Abuse. *The National Household Survey on Drug Abuse,* Rockville, MD, 1988.

"New 800-COCAINE Survey Reports Use of Cocaine or Crack Is Directly Linked to Violence."

"New Jersey's Law Enforcement Community Embraces a New 'Supporting' Role in the War on Drugs."

Page, Jeffrey. "Tracing Lines of Coke to a Sixth-Story Ledge." *The Bergen Record,* Jan. 18, 1990, p. B1.

Pardes, Herbert, Pincus, Harold Alan. "Neuroscience and Psychiatry: An Overview," in *The Integration of Neuroscience and Psychiatry,* Pincus, Harold Alan, Pardes, Herbert, eds. Washington: American Psychiatric Press, 1985, pp. 2–20.

Partnership for a Drug-Free America: Ad, *The New York Times,* Dec. 16, 1989, p. 11.

Paul, Steven M. "Toward the Integration of Neuroscience and Psychiatry," in *The Integration of Neuroscience and Psychiatry,* Pincus, Harold Alan, Pardes, Herbert, eds. Washington: American Psychiatric Press, 1985, pp. 40–52.

"Pennsylvania Workers to Look for Drug Labs." *The New York Times,* Nov. 24, 1989, p. A22.

Pinkney, Deborah S. "Drug-Addicted Newborns Increasing; MDs, Hospitals Face Care Dilemma." *American Medical News,* Feb. 3, 1989, pp. 2, 16.

"Police Chiefs Identify 29 States Enforcing Drug-Free School Zones." Press release, National Association of Chiefs of Police, Aug. 1, 1989.

Porro, Jennifer. "Courts Settle Difficult Questions Regarding Workplace Drug Testing." *Occupational Health and Safety,* Nov. 1989, p. 48, 50.

Posey, Mike. "I Did Drugs Until They Wore Me Out. Then I Stopped [Editorial]." *The New York Times,* Dec. 15, 1989, p. 38.

Post, Robert M. "The Potential of Neuroscience Research for Clinical Psychiatry," in *The Integration of Neuroscience and Psychiatry,*

Pincus, Harold Alan, Pardes, Herbert, eds. Washington: American Psychiatric Press, 1985, pp. 21–38.

PRIDE: The PRIDE Questionnaire For Grades 6–12 National Database 1988–89. Atlanta: PRIDE Inc., 1989.

"Project TRUST Helps Students at Palmetto Junior High School." *Schools Without Drugs: The Challenge,* Mar./Apr. 1989, p. 11.

Psychiatric News, "DSM-IV Multi-Site Field Trials to Compare Proposed Diagnostic Criteria." December 7, 1990, p. 4.

Psychiatric News, "Comorbidity Rates of Substance Abuse, Mental Illness Found to be Surprisingly High." December 21, 1990, p. 2.

Raczynski, James M, Wiebe, Deborah J, Milby, Jesse B., Gurwitch, Robin H. "Behavioral Assessment of Narcotic Detoxification Fear." *Addictive Behaviors,* Vol. 13 (1988), pp. 165–169.

Razavi, Rebecca H. "Be Smart! Campaign Gets New Look." *Schools Without Drugs: The Challenge.* Sept./Oct. 1989, p. 12.

"Reports of Congenital Syphilis Rise." *The New York Times,* Dec. 12, 1989, p. C12.

Ribadeneira, Diego. "Ex-Navy Pilot Fires Drug Warning at Pupils." *The Boston Globe,* Nov. 15, 1989, pp. 31, 34.

Risher-Flowers, Debra, Adinoff, Bryon, Avitz, Bernard, et al. "Circadian Rhythms of Cortisol During Alcohol Withdrawal." *Advances in Alcohol and Substance Abuse,* Vol. 7, No. 3/4 (1988), pp. 37–39.

Robertson, Nan. *Getting Better: Inside Alcoholics Anonymous.* New York: Fawcett Crest, 1988.

Roehrich, Herb, Gold, Mark S. "Emergency Presentations of Crack Abuse." *Emergency Medical Services,* Sep. 1988, pp. 41–44.

Roehrich, Herb, Gold, Mark S. "800-COCAINE: Origin, Significance, and Findings." *The Yale Journal of Biology and Medicine,* 1988; Vol. 61 (1988), pp. 149–155.

Roman, Paul M. "Stuck in the Bottle's Blur." *Employee Assistance,* Oct. 1989, pp. 54–55.

Rome, Howard P. "Editorial Reflections." *Psychiatric Annals,* May 1989, p. 232.

Rome, Howard P. "The Implications of Substance Abuse." *Psychiatric Annals,* April 1986, pp. 203–204.

Rosenthal, A. M. "How Much Is a Baby Worth? [Editorial]." *The New York Times,* Dec. 15, 1989, p. A39.

Rynearson, Edward K. "Personal Reflections: The Bunkhouse." *Psychiatric Annals,* May 1989, pp. 233–234.

Saunders, Marguerite T. "Alcohol Can Be a Dead End for Teen-agers [Letter to the Editor]." *The New York Times,* Nov. 7, 1989.

Schnoll, Sidney H., Daghestani, Amin N. "Treatment of Marijuana Abuse." *Psychiatric Annals,* April 1986, pp. 249–254.

Schuckit, Marc A. "Familial Alcoholism. *Vista Hill Foundation Drug Abuse and Alcoholism Newsletter,* Nov. 1989, pp. 1–4.

Schuckit, Marc A. "Suicidal Behavior and Substance Abuse." *Drug Abuse and Alcoholism Newsletter.* Oct. 1989, pp. 1–3.

Schuster, Charles R. "Consequences of Teenage Drug Use: An Update." *Schools Without Drugs: The Challenge,* Mar./Apr. 1989, pp. 3–6.

Schwartz, Richard H., Gruenewald, Paul J., Klitzner, Michael, Fedio, Paul. "Short-Term Memory Impairment in Cannabis-Dependent Adolescents." *AJDC,* Oct. 1989, pp. 1214–1219.

Searching for Drug-Free School Zones. Press release, National Association of Chiefs of Police, Aug. 1, 1989.

Seymour, Richard, Smith, David E. *The Physician's Guide to Psychoactive Drugs.* New York: The Haworth Press, 1987.

Siegel, Ronald K. "Cocaine Smoking Disorders: Diagnosis and Treatment." *Psychiatric Annals,* Oct. 1984, pp. 728–732.

Smolowe, Jill. "The Drug Thugs." *Time,* May 7, 1988, pp. 28–37.

"Some War. Meanwhile, Crack Undermines America [Editorial]." *The New York Times,* Sept. 24, 1989, p. E24.

Stapleton, J. M., Eckardt, M. J, Martin, P., et al. "Treatment of Alcohol Organic Brain Syndrome with the Serotonin Reuptake Inhibitor Fluvoxamine: A Preliminary Study." *Advances in Alcohol and Substance Abuse,* Vol. 7, No. 3/4 (1988), pp. 47–51.

"State's School Districts Launch 'Total War' on Drugs." *School Safety and Security Management,* Feb. 1989, pp. 12–15.

"Steroids Mean Trouble [Poster]." *Schools Without Drugs: The Challenge.* Sep./Oct. 1989, p. 14.

Stewart, Sally Ann. "Pot Harvest Sets Record." *USA Today,* Oct. 31, 1989, p. 3A.

Stipp, David. "Probing the Human Brain's Functions." *The Wall Street Journal,* Nov. 1, 1989, p. B1.

Stone, Robert. "A Higher Horror of the Whiteness." *Harper's Magazine,* Dec. 1989, pp. 49–54.

"Student Survey Finds Disconcerting Familiarity with Drugs." *Newark* (New Jersey) *Star-Ledger,* Dec. 17, 1989, p. 80.

Suburban Crack Use on the Rise: New Data Shows a Return of the

Upscale Drug Abuser. Fair Oaks Hospital press release, July 22, 1989.

"Surgeon General's Workshop on Drunk Driving Offers Recommendations for Youth." *Schools Without Drugs: The Challenge.* May/June 1989, p. 10.

"Survey Shows Declining Drug Use Among High School Seniors." *Schools Without Drugs: The Challenge,* Mar./Apr. 1989, pp. 1, 14.

Susswein, Ronald. "Law Enforcement's Role in the War on Drugs." *Schools Without Drugs: The Challenge,* May/June 1989, pp. 7–9.

Sweet, Charles W. "Judge: Time to Legalize Drugs Is Now." *The Bergen Record,* Dec. 17, 1989, p. O4.

Symonds, William C., with Ellis, James E., Flynn-Silver, Julia, Zellner, Wendy B., Garland, Susan B. "Is Business Bungling Its Battle with Booze?" *Business Week,* March 25, 1991, pp. 76–78.

Tennant, Forest S. "The Clinical Syndrome of Marijuana Dependence." *Psychiatric Annals,* April 1986, pp. 225–234.

"Testing Shows Regional Contrasts in the Use of Cocaine by Criminals." *The New York Times,* Nov. 19, 1989, p. 34.

"The Credibility Gap on Drugs [Editorial]." *The New York Times,* Dec. 28, 1989, p. 38.

"Tiny Cocaine Doses Cut Blood Flow to the Heart." *The New York Times,* Dec. 7, 1989.

"Tips for Party Planners." *Schools Without Drugs: The Challenge,* Mar./Apr. 1989, pp. 8–9.

"Tips for Principals." *Schools Without Drugs: The Challenge,* Sep./Oct. 1989, pp. 8–9.

Treaster, Joseph B. "Battle Against Drug Trafficking Is Languishing in South America." *The New York Times,* Jan. 1, 1990, pp. A1, 9.

Turner, Carlton E. "The Cocaine Epidemic and Prevention of Future Drug Epidemics." *Psychiatric Annals* Sept. 1988, pp. 507–512.

223,000 U.S. Students Used Cocaine Weekly in 1988–89 School Year. Press release from PRIDE, Sept. 26, 1989.

U.S. Department of Education. *Drug Prevention Curricula: A Guide to Selection and Implementation.* Office of Educational Research and Improvement, U.S. Department of Education, 1988.

U.S. Department of Education. *What Works: Schools Without Drugs.* U. S. Department of Education, 1989.

U.S. Department of Labor. *What Works: Workplaces Without Drugs.* U.S. Department of Labor (n.d.).

U.S. Department of Labor, Bureau of Labor Statistics. *Survey of Em-*

ployer Anti-Drug Programs. U.S. Department of Labor Report 760, Jan. 1989.

U.S. Department of Justice. *A Special Report on Ice.* U.S. Department of Justice, Drug Enforcement Administration, Office of Intelligence, Oct. 1989.

Van Buren, Abigail. "Why Not Charge Rent for Jail Time?" *The Bergen Record,* Dec. 28, 1989.

Verebey, Karl, Gold, Mark S. "Endorphins and Mental Disease." in *Handbook of Neurochemistry Vol. 10,* Lajtha, Agbel, ed. New York: Plenum Publishing Corporation, 1985, pp. 589–615.

Vereby, Karl, Gold, Mark S. "From Coca Leaves to Crack: The Effects of Dose and Route of Administration in Abuse Liability." *Advances in Alcohol and Substance Abuse,* 8(2): 53–69; 1989.

Verebey, Karl, Gold, Mark S. "From Coca Leaves to Crack: The Effects of Dose and Routes of Administration in Abuse Liability." *Psychiatric Annals,* Sep. 1988, pp. 513–520.

Verebey, Karl, Gold, Mark S., Mule, S. Joseph. "Laboratory Testing in the Diagnosis of Marijuana Intoxication and Withdrawal." *Psychiatric Annals,* April 1986, pp. 235–241.

Vereby, Karl, Martin, David M., Gold, Mark S. "Interpretation of Drug Abuse Testing: Strengths and Limitations of Current Methodology." *Psychiatric Medicine,* Vol. 3, No. 3 (1987), pp. 287–297.

Volkow, Nora D., Swann, Alan C., eds. *Cocaine in the Brain.* New Brunswick, N.J.: Rutgers University Press, 1990.

"War on Drugs Must Begin on the Poverty Front [Letter]." *The New York Times,* Dec. 26, 1989, p. 24.

Washton, Arnold M., Gold, Mark S., eds. *Cocaine: A Clinician's Handbook.* New York: Guilford Press, 1987.

Washton, Arnold M., Gold, Mark S., Pottash, A.L.C. "Opiate and Cocaine Dependencies." *Drug Dependency,* April 1985, pp. 294–300.

Washton, Arnold M., Gold, Mark S., Pottash, A. Carter, Semlitz, Linda. "Adolescent Cocaine Abusers." *The Lancet,* Sept. 29, 1984, p. 746.

Watkins, George T. "Window of Opportunity." *EAP Digest,* Sept./Oct. 1989, p. 6.

Weiss, Roger D., Mirin, Steven M. "The Dual Diagnosis Alcohol: Evaluation and Treatment." *Psychiatric Annals,* May 1989, pp. 261–265.

Wesson, Donald R., Camber, Susan. "Inpatient vs. Outpatient Treatment of the Cocaine-Dependent Individual." (No source).

The White House. *National Drug Control Strategy.* Office of National Drug Control Policy, Sept. 1989 and Feb. 1991.

The White House. *National Drug Control Strategy: Executive Summary.* Office of National Drug Control Policy, Sept. 1989.

The White House Conference for a Drug Free America. *Final Report.* Washington: U.S. Government Printing Office, 1988.

Yandow, Valery. "Alcoholism in Women." *Psychiatric Annals,* May 1989, pp. 243–247.

Yett, Andrew. "All Agree on Failure of Our Drug Strategy [letter]." *The New York Times,* Jan. 1, 1990, p. 24.

Zimberg, Sheldon. "Diagnosis and Management of the Elderly Alcoholic," in *Alcohol and Drug Abuse in Old Age,* Atkinson, Roland M., ed. Washington: American Psychiatric Press, 1984, pp. 24–33.

Zwerling, C., Ryan. J., Orav, E. J., "The Efficacy of Preemployment Drug Screening for Marijuana and Cocaine in Predicting Employment Outcome." *Journal of the American Medical Association,* Nov. 28, 1990. Vol. 26A, no. 20, pp. 2639–43.

INDEX